Lanzarote

To top a volcano's corona and gaze inside is an experience not to be missed and never to be forgotten. Lanzarote may be the most dramatic and exciting venue we have found. Though hot, it is breezy and perfectly comfortable for walking. The landscape is unlike anything in the world and a few minutes walking away from the car is rewarded far more than can possibly be imagined.

> *'It's really fun to be striving to pick out a route to the top of a mountain, or to follow a map, or to decipher the ravings of a walking guide author. The walk is strenuous in places but you don't notice because the barranco is so exciting and the mountain path thrilling and then suddenly you reach the corona and look down in absolute awe into the bowl of a volcano, or you struggle to the peak and get a view of the whole world.'*

Note: *This text is offered on the inventive new 'Createspace' Publishing platform for two reasons:*

1) *The costs to the reader are far lower than traditional publishing houses.*
2) *It is easy to update and improve the work; the text is continually under review. To this end the readers and the authors form a community to develop the work. As a reader, you are invited to email suggestions to nwheeler@brookes.ac.uk Contributions may be simple 'typo' alerts, corrections to detail, new areas to cover, etc. All contributors are acknowledged in the print and E-Book versions, with our thanks.*

ISBN 10 - 1543283977
ISBN 13 - 9781543283976

We are…

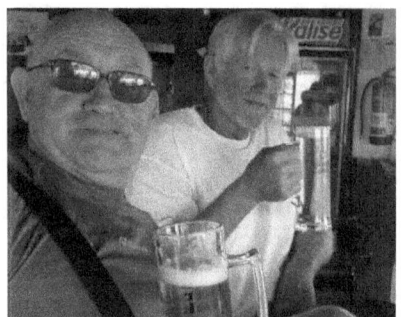

Alan: the brains of the operation; Neil: the chronicler. Alan knows nearly every path on the island and either he accompanies the acolytes or directs the walk from a distance. I put it onto paper.

It always starts in Reiners Bar, with a couple of Estrella *'Dos jarra pour favour.'*

It sometimes goes, *'Be ready at nine, tomorrow, if you can. I've got a walk planned'*. That presages a cracking good outing.

Or else it's, *'Here's a walk you might like'*. That means I'm going alone. Good fun, but I'll get lost.

Then there's Emma. She accompanies whenever she can, mostly because she thinks Neil shouldn't be allowed out alone. I expect she's right; she usually is. And Wendy, whose blog and kindness have made everything possible.

ISBN 10 - 1543283977

ISBN 13 - 9781543283976

First published 2017

Lambert, A and Wheeler, N. (2017) *Walking in Lanzarote*. Slough: Createspace publishing.

Contents

Join us…

For our first five years visiting Lanzarote I believed that lying on a sun-bed was of itself exhausting enough and to arise and walk to the pool was a heroic achievement worthy of universal approbation.

Walking for any distance was right out!

For the last few years, though, I've found that that is not so. Egged on by Alan I've walked up endless mountains and marvelled at island views and the insides of volcanoes. The view from some of the cliffs and coronas is breath-taking *(although, admittedly that could just be the walk to reach them)*. A side effect of this exercise is that it has resolved the problem of dampness in my wardrobe. Previously, I found that the trousers I wore to fly to Lanzarote would shrink in the wardrobe and prove too small to wear for the return trip; the wardrobes must be damp. Since I started walking, I have found the *'shrinking in the wardrobe'* problem wholly alleviated. Sometimes they are too big! Bring a belt.

I do not imagine myself learned with regard to Lanzarote after fewer than ten years. But I do know a man who is. Alan has been my walking mentor in person and by remote instruction for some good time.

This guide reports on Alan's instruction and my slow learning journey to progressively understand and appreciate an island that has me completely captivated. If you use it you will not learn from me, but you might just learn something with me. As I observe and wonder, I enquire and find out. If you walk with me, we will be discovering Lanzarote together. I hope that you will.

The Old Man of the Hills   &   Emma

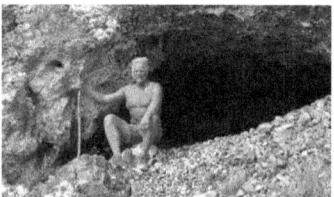   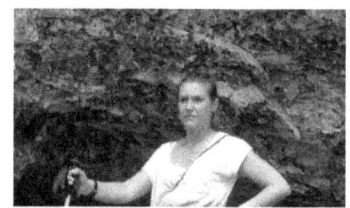

On walking guides…

Walking guides come in many forms, and it is *'horses for courses'.* Some are written by professional writers who have been granted enough expenses for a week in a resort and write excellent prose about their limited 'finds'. This will suit the short-visit tourist adequately but walks tend to be basic, without the little diversions that make them exciting. Another model is the *'back-of-my-hand'* local enthusiast who will know every twisty turn, diversion and staggering view in the locality and describe them for you as well as he/she can. This well suits the adventurous walker who wants the best and doesn't mind deciphering opaque explanations and still getting lost. When you know something very well it's easy to assume rather than explain. Some fine guides endeavour to combine both, in a rich compromise.

This guide is certainly not better or worse than those approaches; it's just different. It will suit some readers. The intention is for the reader to explore a fantastic island alongside the author. As I discover, I report so that you can find it, too. You might learn about Lanzarote alongside me, but not from me.

And roughly speaking, as a guide, anything in italics can be skipped over – probably best that you do.

On litter…

Self-evidently, walkers enjoy and respect the countryside and do not leave litter, so this book does not exhort you to *'take it home'.* However, for myself I go one step further. It is my practice to take 4-cent carrier bag on every walk and set myself the target of filling it with cans, bottles and plastics before the end of the walk. Sadly, this is not a difficult challenge. Patently, one old chap with a carrier bag will not make a dent in Lanzarote's litter problem, but it is good to feel that you left it better than you found it if only slightly. As guests in an unbelievable landscape perhaps it behoves us to make a positive contribution, be it never so small.

On safety...

I don't really like heights, but I walk up mountains and down cliffs. If vertigo is an issue for you *(as it is for me)*, it might be because of the odd perspective you get from and each level seeming to move differently as you walk. This is a problem of parallax.

I'm a height wimp, so I find it good to watch my feet when walking and stand dead still when I want to admire the view.

Winds can be extreme on Lanzarote and it is radically varied on different parts of the island. On occasion we have decided not to get out of the car at all, so badly was it rocking in the wind. All mountain peak, corona or cliff walks should be seen as *out-of-bounds* on a windy day.

Don't run out of light. Dusk this near the equator is brief; it goes dark fast! So check the sundown time and allow a big margin for error when planning an outing.

All of these walks have been extensively tested; we find them safe enough – for us. By the time you read it, things can have changed, because of rain, rock falls, erosion or whatever. And your agility might be different from ours, so you must judge the safety of every enterprise you undertake. We are not saying that any walk is safe today or for you, only that it was safe when we did it, for us.

We will not accept responsibility for misfortune that occurs on your walk. You walk at your own risk!

And health...

This walking lark is worth it for the breath-taking views but to make it healthy they recon you need to be a little breathless on the ascents but still able to hold a conversation. *(Mind you that last bit always looks a bit dodgy when I walk alone.)* Carry sun block and lip-balm for regular application, especially if you're not well thatched. Carry copious water. Sometimes I don't get thirsty at all and the next time, a litre is gone in no time. Possibly we are affected by humidity. When the air is very dry and whipping past on a hot day it does seem to rip the moisture out of you.

Blisters happen, so carry plasters. I also carry a spare pair of shoes and socks, as different from the ones I am walking in as possible. That means that if a shoe is rubbing I can put on another pair that does not have the same pressure points. Wear sun protecting clothes.

A compass and map will get you home wherever you are and a whistle is good in the event that you want to attract attention. Signal is pretty good so take a 'phone and know where you are should you need to summon aid. There is only one really good map: *'Lanzarote Tour and Trail'*. It's not in many shops here so Google it!

On paths...

We use the term 'path' rather loosely in places. Some are thin but clear; sometimes they vanish without warning. I find that if the path vanishes, it's because I've wondered off it. If I stop and look around I usually spot it and return is easy. Sometimes it just peters out. Then it is good to have Hiawatha with you; if you can see trainer prints every now and then you are probably still on the route.

Sometimes you realise that it is not a path, but a goat trail; sometimes it is a rain gulley (Barranco).

There are also *'Hogwarts paths'* that can be clear as day from a distance but when you reach them and try to follow them, they will completely vanish. Lanzarote *'Hogwart's paths'* appear and disappear at will. I personally think that they do so simply to inconvenience walkers. For more on this, see Appendix 3

Jerome K Jerome says of kettles, 'one must pretend to take no notice of it, if you want it to boil. It is a good plan, too, to talk loudly about how you don't feel like tea and will not drink any of it when it's ready and would really prefer lemonade.'

I find the same works for some paths. If I say 'Pick path A' or 'Take track B' you will not find either in a month of weekends. If we pretend not to care about paths at all, then one will pop up in no time. Just until it thinks you are beginning to like following it and then it will instantly vanish. I tried a good trick on one. When I stumbled upon it I turned and followed it backwards for that way it was as clear as day. The path was happy to be followed as long as it thought it was leading me in the wrong direction. Before long it smelled a rat, though, and realized that I was liking following it so 'Poof!' it was gone.

So, like Jerome, we give out that we do not want to use the path anyway. One day we are on a 'path unlooked for' and we follow it for a bit loudly saying things like, 'I'm not bothered about this path either way. Are you, Emma?' 'No not me; I'm happy keeping the mountain on my left elbow; don't need a path at all, really. Aren't you the same, Neil?' 'Oh, yes, that's good enough for me; I've no use for a path.' Keeping this up means that the path continues for some way before it cottons on to our ruse and then 'Poof!' It is Gone.

Anyway, each walk is independently pilot tested to assure me that the description works, so you should be OK, and even if you are unable to find a trail (maybe it was washed away) it's a small island and a road always appears before long.

On equipment...

A compass and a map make a good start. That way, you'll find a route under any circumstances. More importantly, when you reach a peak, you're surrounded by views over a range of villages, mountains and whatnot and it is great fun to sit and identify each from the map. There is only one really good map:

'Lanzarote Tour and Trail'. It's not in many shops here, so Google it!

Some people like to walk in heavy hiking boots, but for most of these walks, walking trainers are enough. Only where walking is over very rocky lava would a hard sole be advisable to prevent meta-tarsal bruising. The walk guide will warn you.

I take spare footwear, as different from what I have on my feet as possible. If I get a blister, I can change into something with different pressure points. Sandals, for instance mean that blistered toes are safe.

Water is crucial. Decide how much you need for the number of hours that you will walk and double it. On some occasions, when the wind is strong and the humidity very low, water loss can be quite remarkable. An ice cold beer is recommended in many of the walks but that's not always the best way to re-hydrate. Take plenty of water before starting on the Estrella.

Take sun cream for periodic reapplying and protective headwear, *(especially if you are folically challenged as is one of the authors)*.

A stick has two benefits.

> Firstly, on some walks the ground is unsteady because gravel and stones can move underfoot. A third point of contact can be a life-saver when the ground slips and your feet go out from under you. My stick has saved me on many occasions.

> Secondly, in terms of exercise value, using a stick is an upper limb workout to complement your lower limb exercise. Alternate hands and you will develop muscle evenly.

Just occasionally, you might be pleased that have lightweight raingear in your backpack. When it rains in Lanzarote, it doesn't mess around!

Flora and fauna

Far more grows on the island than people imagine; the soil is very much more fertile that it appears and water can be taken from the humid atmosphere by cunning deployment of pecon. Farming includes: Lanzarote palms, grapes, figs, olives, orange, lemon, almonds, potatoes, leeks, onions, peas, strawberries, melons, chillies and peppers, etc *(and etc!)*. The fresh food offer with minimal food miles is quite remarkable.

Wild plants include a wealth of cacti, geraniums, sedum, nicotiana, and many more. After a little rain, the island hosts masses of wild-flower meadows.

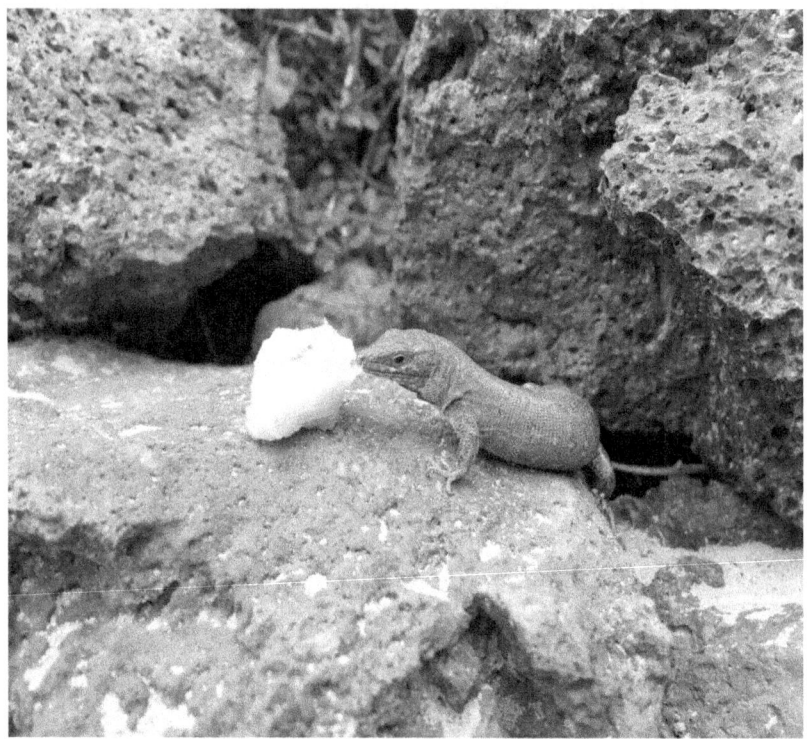

In the sky, there are hawks, kestrels, buzzards, ravens, little egrets, choughs, sparrows, hoopoes, doves, pipits, chaffinches, goldcrests, canaries and more.

On the ground there are lizards and their heavier cousins, geckoes. These will eat banana from your hand in many of the beachside pods. There are mice, rabbits and hedgehogs everywhere if you look for the signs.

In the sea there is an incredible array of fish.

Places to visit

For us, the island is unrivalled in the world for landscape and artefacts and it rewards a trip out by car when you are showing the unquestionable wisdom of declining to walk up a mountain. The following is a basic list and we generally don't like visitors to leave until they have experienced each of them at least once. As an economy, it is possible to buy a batch of tickets allowing entry to five of these remarkable locations at a significant reduction – and well worth it.

The Cactus Garden.

Guatiza on the LZ1 hosts this amazing garden. The layout is extremely clever and the collection of cacti breath-taking. A look inside the windmill is also a privilege. Nearby, in Mala, there is the renowned Arepera Restaurant and across the main road from there it is possible to see *(from the road and for free)* an almost better cactus garden; check out both on one trip.

Jamos Del Aqua.

This staggering cave system is on the LZ1 Orzola Road is a most amazing experience, not to be missed, but frequently to be repeated *(we do, anyway)*.

Cueva los Verda.

Another cave system, actually linked to Jamos *Del Aqua,* being part of the same lava tube, is just off the LZ1 Orzola road on the LZ204. This is a very different but equally amazing experience, also not to be missed.

The Mirador Del Rio.

This Mirador (viewing point) is near Orzola on the North-West extreme of the island and is a magnificent Cesar Monrique construction. After enjoying the building and the view for a bit, I have to marvel at the engineers who built it.

Salinas de Janubio

On the South-West coast, not far from Playa Blanca is an active salt pan, where hills of salt are to be seen. There is an intriguing system of canals designed to take sea water and fill each bay where it is left to evaporate and the salt collected by hand. This pan is still said to produce 15,000 tonnes of salt per year, but that is less than a third of production of this industry in its heyday. Before, refrigeration, the salt was a major industry for the island, being used to preserve fish. Today's harvest is exported. *(There being little need to salt the roads in Lanzarote.)*

Fuego de Timanfaya.

The famous, Fire Mountain, on the west of the island is a true spectacle. Ideally visit at opening time (10-am) because the access is narrow and traffic builds up later in the day. The crust is thin and ground too hot in places to walk. See geysers, barbeque meat over the hot ground and take the bus tour over a landscape that you will never forget.

Los Hevidaros

This is a fabulous spectacle on the West coast, on the LZ702 that sees crashing waves assault the cliff and pass under natural arches and you can watch it all from walkways and galleries built into and on top of the cliff. This is unlike anything else on the island. Like so much else that is good on Lanzarote the layout was designed by Cesar Monrique.

El Golfo.

On the West coast, on the LZ702 lies this is a charming village and a short walk *(No, Really; it is a very short walk)* over a hill takes you to an emerald green inland lake. There are a few nice restaurants, too.

The two homes of Cesar Monrique,

Both of Monrique's homes were donated to become museums. One is in Haria and the other (The Foundation) is near to Tahiche. Both need to be seen *(to be believed)*. They represent eccentricity at its most brilliant.

Lag Omar,

In Nazaret near Teguise, signed from the LZ10, Lag Omar is a home built by Cesar Monrique for Omar Sharif. It is set into a quarry rock face with external staircases linking normal rooms, each build into a cave. The surreal placing of (for example) modern kitchen fittings into a cave is something that will blow you away.

Castillo Santa Barbara

Is a castle near to the old capital town, Teguise, where it was once necessary to retreat from pirates; a dramatic building with far reaching views. A few minutes' study here will give a real insight into the lives of islanders plagued by pirates.

Wine and cheese, unspoiled Bodega

Leaving Orzola heading South-Westerly on the LZ201, you may be lucky enough to see a hand painted sign on your right for this Mexican style farm. Drive in for charming wine and cheese tasting in a building that might be a living museum. This is much more 'real' (*not to say cheaper*) than the big commercial wineries that you would find in La Garia.

Lanzarote a Caballo

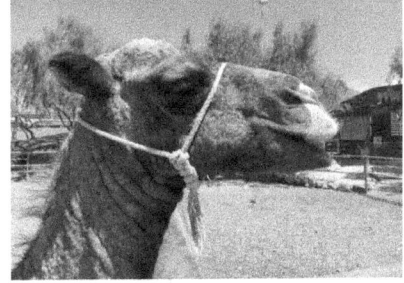

To be found on the LZ2 near Playa del Carmen the Lanzarote a Caballo offers pony and camel riding in a very nice and informal way. You can ride camels at the Fuego de Timanfaya, but that is a little *coach-trippy*. For a far more personal experience riding on

15

a saddle not in a basket, go to Cabello. If you prefer, they would arrange horse riding, buggies, trikes, and even paint ball *(if you must).* 10:00 AM to 05:30 PM.

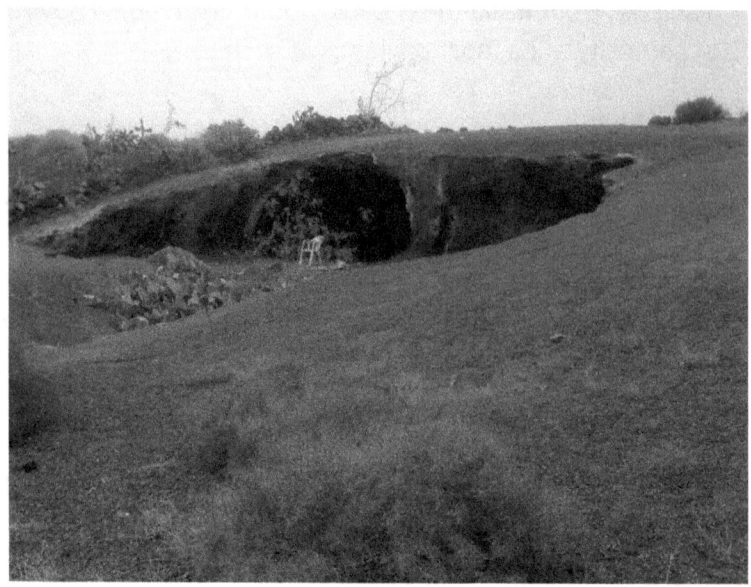

Beaches

Playa de Papagayo, near Playa Blanca is a great place to play in the waves on a sandy beach and affords plenty of scope for sandcastles. One beach is clothed; one beach is naturist. You can take your pick.

Playa de Famara on the West coast is a long sandy beach great for views and sun with a naturist tolerance, but although there are surfers galore, it is not recommended for swimming as the currents are dangerous and drownings are recorded almost every year.

Orzola and Isla Graciosa. At the northern extremity of the island, on the LZ1 Orzola has the ferry to Isla Graciosa which has some very fine beaches. Heading North on the LZ1, approaching Orzola there are several small isolated sandy places by the water with parking allowing secluded bathing and Orzola itself has a good safe beach.

Towns

See: Haria, Teguise, Yaiza, Uga and Femes if nowhere else, but really the style of house and their general unspoiled nature makes all of the old towns a treat to visit.

(The new ones, of course, are a matter of taste.)

Markets

Arrecife   **Monday to Friday:**
Recova Market 9am to 2pm - Fresh local produce and local artisan craft shops
Fish Market - 9am to 1pm - Local fish and sea food caught fresh each day

Playa Blanca   **Wednesday & Saturday**
Marina Rubicon - 9.30am to 1.30pm - About 30 stalls with crafts, jewellery, arts and books

Costa Teguise   **Friday**
Pueblo Marinero - 6pm to 10pm - Small and busy evening market, mainly crafts and souvenirs, great atmosphere.

Haria   **Saturday**
Artisan Market - 10am to 2.30pm - Various stalls with handmade crafts and artwork, some local produce stalls, a bit quirky and different.

Tias   **Saturday**
Recova Market - 9am to 2pm - Small market with local goods and produce

Mancha Blanca   **Sunday**
Local agricultural market- 9am to 2pm - The best island market for local produce and fresh fruit and vegetables.

Teguise   **Sunday**
Island market - 9am to 2pm - The biggest market in Lanzarote selling everything; arts, jewellery, clothes, bags, linen and leather goods.

Notes

Las Calderas, circular walk from Charco Del Palo

This is a 3-hour, trainers, walk, moderately strenuous, with only minimal risk of vertigo, in spite of a 216m peak height. Fabulous views. Best sighting of a volcano on the island!

Take a compass, binoculars, a map and your stick.

Some walks take us over well-trodden paths where your heart-attack will see you discovered and revived in mere minutes. We love this one, though, because it takes us on *the path less Travelled*

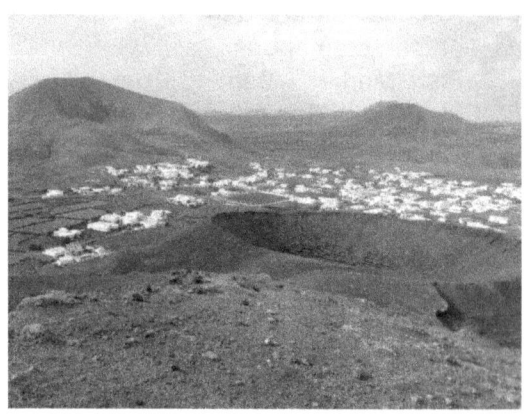

(Frost,1920) and when you are eventually found it will be no more than your bleached bones that remain to decorate the scenery.

Set out from the south end of Charco Del Palo, taking the jeep track up towards the mountain. Swing right and observe cairns on the hilltop to the right. Unlike many, these appear to be completely gratuitous. If you fancy an extra 2-minute climb, there is an excellent view back over Charco from these cairns. Ahead we soon see the paired mountains: Colorada and Mojon which give their named to Charco Del Palo roads.

This walk is worth it for the breath-taking views, but to make it healthy, I recon you need to be a little breathless on the ascents but still able to hold a conversation. Mind you that last bit always looks a bit dodgy if I walk alone.

The track continues towards a ruined farmhouse, which must have once been a glorious location overlooking the sea and the village, but long since abandoned. Shortly before that landmark we branch off to follow a track on the left.

This track continues, until on both sides of the road farmers quarry Pecon, to be spread on the fields where they condense dew from moisture rich winds and trickle it onto crops.

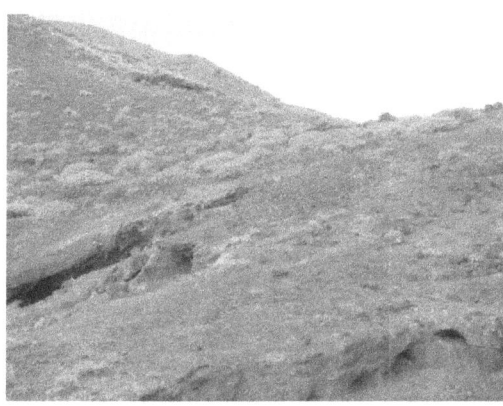

In the left-side quarry is a nice small cave, which in England would be fully equipped and rented out as a 'hobbit hole' for £50/night.

To the right of the road is a faint jeep track, which we follow between two more quarries to a gateway in the wall up ahead.

Through the gateway we turn a little to the left and follow the spine/ridge to the right of two more hobbit holes (OK, Lava tunnels). By the higher of these two hobbit holes there is a path off to the right. Ignore this for the present. It will be our way back, later.

We proceed breathlessly ever-upwards until we suddenly find ourselves on the corona of our volcano. OK, it is not much of a path. ('*You dimwit, you've got us lost again, haven't you?*') For me, it is enough to say *just keep going upwards*. The reader must decide.

Standing on the corona's edge, to the left is a fine view of the sea, overlooking Charco Del Palo and Los Cocoteros. Behind us, we can see Mala, Arrieta, Punta Mujeres and Jamos Del Agua. To the right is the basin of the volcano, which has been extensively farmed in the past. It is very inviting, but this is not the easy way to reach it. That will come later.

Following the corona around is easy, it is smooth and wide and the slope on either side is relatively innocent. Interestingly, as the path goes higher, rather than the barren rocks we might expect, the ground becomes quite lush and green. Many of the volcano tops do this. Struggling up over barren rocks and pecon paths, we often find a quite lush green area opens up ahead of us. Volcanic tops can prove to be far more verdant than their lower slopes.

Reaching the concrete Trig point (216 metres above our start point) it is about an hour from the start.

From here there is an astonishing view, over Guatiza to Montana Tinamala and Montana Guenla in the foreground and between them in the distance we can see all of the way to a fabulous array of mountains in the distant National park.

With a good map, we are able to put a name to a good many of these peaks. Scanning to the right we can see the golf ball and wind farm on the ridge.

More exciting than all of that, though, is the view down onto the top of probably the most complete volcanic corona on the island. *(Our Alan explains that the coronas are usually lopsided because of the effect of prevailing winds on the ash deposits. That is why most of the volcanoes slope in the same direction.)* This one does not slope at all, possibly because it is protected from wind by its bigger brothers on all sides. It is just fabulous to see it from above like this.

We follow the corona further around and head towards a second peak ahead of us. That, *there are many roads up the mountain'* is very evident here, so we can pick any route to the second peak that we like and enjoy the view further around to the North. *En route* to the second high point we can recognise a saddle between the two peaks, and observe a nice Hobbit Hole, with a rough wall protecting the entrance, formerly used as a tool store.

At the lowest point of the saddle between these two peaks there is a gulley (barranco) and to the left of that is a good path that takes us to the *small-but-perfectly-formed* volcano, already admired. We take a walk around this second, lower corona. Some paths look easy and when we attempt them prove extremely intimidating *(You're a total ****wit; you're going to get us killed; etc)*. Others look difficult and then prove to be quite easy. This is one of the latter types. The corona looks difficult at first but when you walk it is really quite easy. Oddly we find clockwise easier than anticlockwise *(and we're not even catholic)*. If vertigo is an issue, it might be because of the odd perspective you get from each level moving differently as you walk. It is a parallax problem. I'm a height wimp, so I find it good to watch my feet when walking and stand dead still when I want to admire the view.

Although the corona is complete, there are two slightly lower points and at each there is a rough path down into the volcanic bowl. This extra climb is well worth the little bit of extra effort involved.

Having visited the floor of this volcano, we go to the North side of the corona where we see a path that winds through a landslip/quarry, down to Guatiza. Behind us as we descend is a veritable Shire of hobbit houses.

Reaching the town, we walk onto the tarmac road and follow it around to the right. We keep turning right with the mountain always on our right shoulder, passing potato fields and cactus fields until we slowly move onto rougher tarmac and leave the settlement behind us.

To our left we soon find a turning that would take us to the Arepera, and a cold beer, at the cost of 10-mins each way, if you want, as long as it is after 1.30, Tuesday - Sunday. The next road on the left is a private lane to a farm, with an interesting al jibe (cistern) made out of a volcanic cave.

Shortly after this there is a jeep track on our right. We could continue along the rough tarmac road to the ruined farm and thence home, or if we have any sense of adventure left in us, follow this jeep track to the right. This track ends and there are two paths. One on a wall to our left is a dead end; we take the one to the right. This is faint but just visible. To our right we see that we are looking down into a volcanic basin, nicely terraced, with a stair down to the floor and an abandoned building.

Having admired the basin, we follow the path as best we can and will be coming around the mountain (♫...when she comes♫). Suddenly we will see the ridge we climbed up so long ago and so very unwisely. The path will lead us on until we realise that we are stood in another volcanic basin. Across, on the next mountain, we can clearly see the path that we will

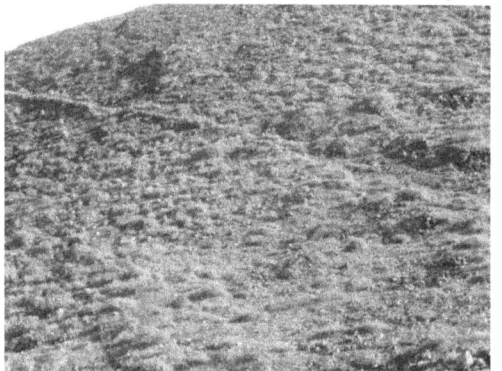

follow to take us back to the hobbit hole we passed on the hill. We note this path carefully, because when we come to try to follow it we will find it has become totally invisible and finding it is an act of faith. With or without

this last path we are following the contour around to the higher of the hobbit houses on the hill that we noted earlier. From here we walk down the slope, between the quarries, back to the 'road' and home (at last! Vowing never to walk

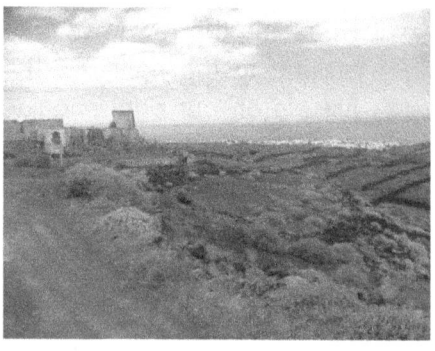

again, but knowing that it is an addiction not easily cured).

Charco Del Palo & Mala: Sand and Volcano Basin Loop

This is a 3-hour, trainers, walk, not at all strenuous, with no risk of vertigo. Pleasant views of the sea, Mala town and volcano. A good walk for a windy day when mountains are not a possibility.

Remote in places. Some walks take us over well-trodden paths where your heart-attack will see you discovered and revived in mere minutes. We love this one, though, because it takes us on *the path less Travelled* (Frost,1920) so when you are eventually

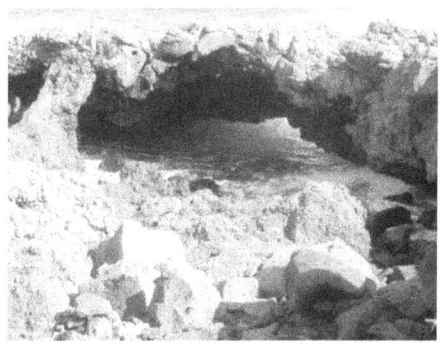

found it may be no more than your sun-bleached bones that remain to decorate the scenery .

Take your stick.

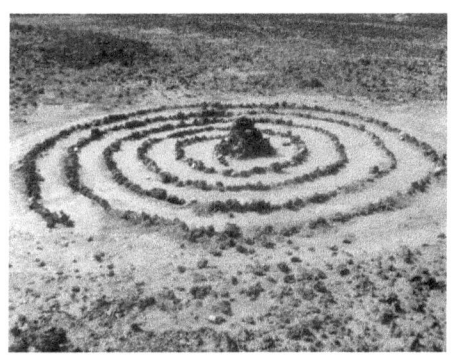

We leave Charco heading north up the coast. The path is clear enough winding over sand and lava. The cliff is not high, but dramatic in places and if there's any wind expect spray.

Look out for stone designs and pods, everywhere. The spiral maze is popular on the island. *Sometimes called a Celtic Maze, mazes have been found all over the world as far back as 3,500 BC. Purpose is unknown, but originally religious and more recently to walk them has been described as a form of meditation.* Anyway, we walk past a remote home, and the ubiquitous half-built house, and eventually, after nearly an hour reach a pleasant little man-made swimming bay. Mala's beach

Lanzarote's celebrated *'Don't do anything at all'* sign applies.

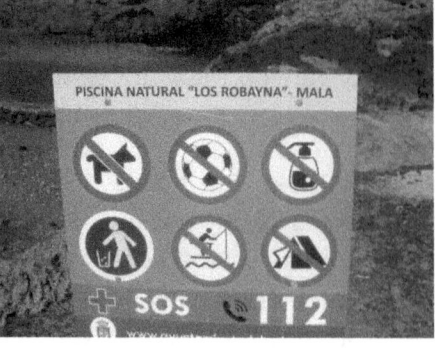

We retrace our steps a very little to find a rough road heading inland passing a couple of nice villas. The path reaches a tar macadam road and not

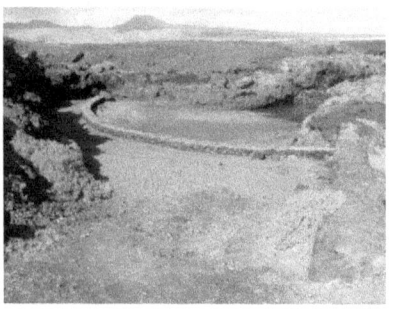

wanting that, we turn Left. We go clockwise around a fine house with a dramatic wall before passing a few very nice gardens.

We reach a T-junction and turn Right, and go straight across a cross-road to come to a power tower. Left past the tower, we eventually emerge at The Cantina Restaurant which is Mala's Sociodad. We might be served a cold beer here, or wait for the Arepera. If it is morning, then the restaurants are closed but we can turn Left on the high street where Pedro's Supermercado keep beer in a cooler until they close at 1pm. Opposite Pedro's, on the Left is a Pharmacia, should the walk have given you blisters.

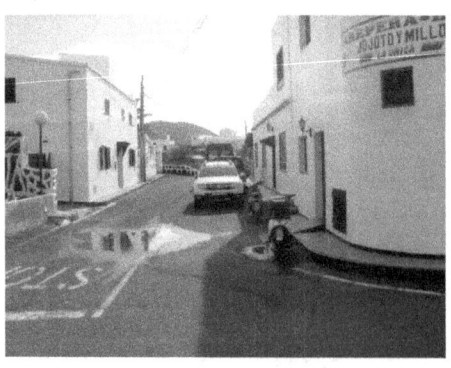

We turn Left after the Pharmacia and ahead, like an oasis, we can see The Arepera. They sell beer so cold that there are ice crystals in the froth.

We take the road on the left of The Arepera. Then, like English politics, we turn Left and then rapidly swing to the Right.

In the road, notice a rough concrete hump to channel water. This takes rain off the road to fill an al jibe that can be seen just over the wall.

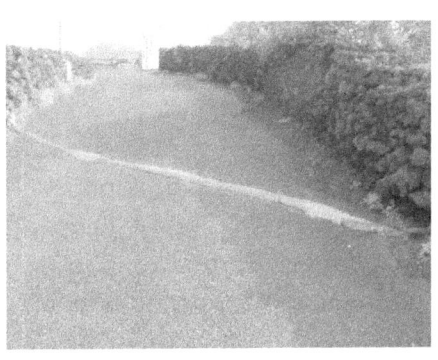

The track continues for 20-mins until reaching a T-junction, where we turn Left, for home. After 250-metres, there is a jeep track on the Right. If you wanted you could keep on the tarmac road here and it would return you to Charco – nobody would think less of you. If you have any spirit left in you, and have not consumed more than one jarra, then take the path on the Right. It continues for a short while and then ends. There are two paths evident. A high one on the Left is a cul-de-sac. We take the faint one on the Right. To our right we see that we are overlooking a volcano basin, cultivated and with a path down to a ruined building. Pop down if you wish.

Our path continues, alongside the highest of the terrace walls and we round the mountain to see that we are in another volcano basin.

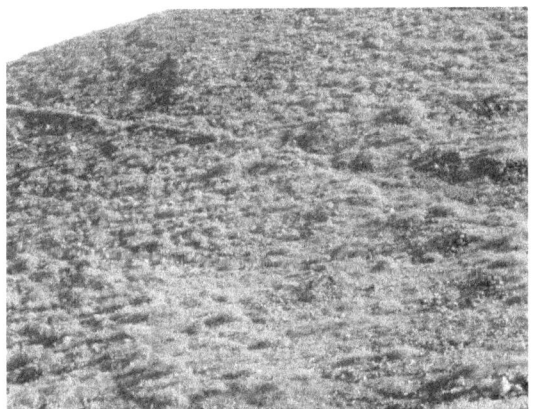

The path around the next mountain is plain to see. But mark it closely, because when we try to follow it will completely vanish. Don't take your eyes off it!

Having finally found and followed the Hogwarts vanishing path, we come out at a hole in the mountain, which looks rough but includes a very nice hobbit hole if you look. We, carefully walk down the mountain, passing another hobbit hole and crossing a wall pass between two quarries. Noticing two piles of stone, clearly put there, but we ponder *how* and more importantly *why* they did that.

We pass through a gap in the wall and follow a faint vehicle track down until it joins a slightly better one by a pair of quarries. Turn left and follow until it reaches a T-junction. Left is the landmark ruined farm and Right is home.

Reaching Charco, we seek out our post-perambulatory cold beer and self-deprecatory conversations. Why **do** we do it?

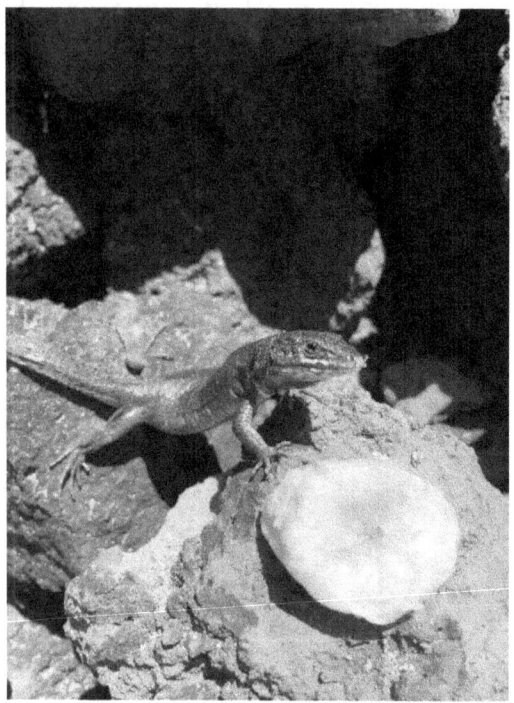

Notes

This is a 1½-hour, trainers, walk, not very strenuous, with no real risk of vertigo, and gets you into the basin of the volcano which is nice. Odd stretches are for the intrepid, but not that bad!

Take a compass, binoculars and a map and your stick.

Some walks take us over well-trodden paths where your heart-attack will see you discovered and revived in mere minutes. We love this one because it takes us on *the path less Travelled* (Frost,1920) and when you are eventually found it will be no more than your bleached bones that remain to decorate the scenery.

Set out from the south end of Charco Del Palo, taking the jeep 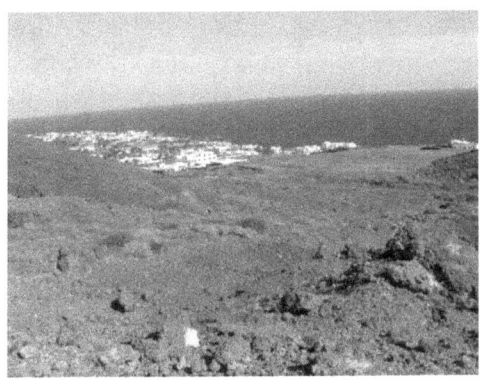 track up towards the mountain. Swing right and observe cairns on the hilltop to the right. Unlike many, these appear to be completely gratuitous. If you fancy an extra 2-minute climb, there is an excellent view back over Charco from these cairns.

Ahead we soon see the paired mountains: Colorada and Mojon which give their named to Charco Del Palo roads.

 The track continues to pass a ruined farmhouse, which must have once been a glorious location overlooking the sea and the village, but long since abandoned. Shortly before the climb to that landmark we branch off to follow a track on the left. We do not go to the ruin, but you might like to detour up and admire the view they used to have. Then, back down to the fork in the road.

This new track continues, North, until on both sides of the road farmers quarry Pecon, to be spread on the fields where they condense dew from moisture rich winds and trickle it onto crops. In the left-side quarry is a nice little cave, which in England would be fully equipped and rented out as a 'hobbit hole' for £50/night.

To the right of the road is a very faint jeep track, which we follow between two more quarries to a gateway in the wall above us. *OK you would not want to take a jeep up this 'track'; neither would I. But these islanders are made of sterner stuff. To see the places they can take a lorry can be a most wondrous sight indeed.*

Through the gateway, over a low wall and we turn a little to the left to follow the spine/ridge to the right of two more hobbit holes (OK, Lava tunnels). At the second, higher, hole it is nice to rest, eat and imbibe, while removing pecon from our more intimate garments. Looking down over the valley, this dwelling has a fabulous view and we can clearly see the jeep track that we were so scornful about earlier. By the higher of these two hobbit holes there is a path off to the right. We follow this path as best we can. It is one of those Hogwarts that sometimes likes to become invisible. After a few minutes we cross a dry stream and realise that we are standing in the basin of the volcano. These volcanic basins are just fabulous to experience. This one has been cultivated in the past, but no more. Gaze all around *(stand and rotate through 360-deg)* and then look up at the volcano corona and thank your lucky stars that we did not choose the walk that takes us to the mountain top.

The path *(and we use the term loosely)* continues around the mountain and soon we find ourselves coming out onto a Jeep track. Here we are standing looking down at a second volcano basin. This is also well cultivated, with paths down over the terraces to the basin and a little hut. That might be enough to entice us to pop down and back up before continuing along the jeep track.

The track ends in a T-junction. If we turn Right it will return us to the ruined farm and thence home! If we turn Left and then take the second road on our Right it will take us to the Arepera and the best cold beer on the island. This out 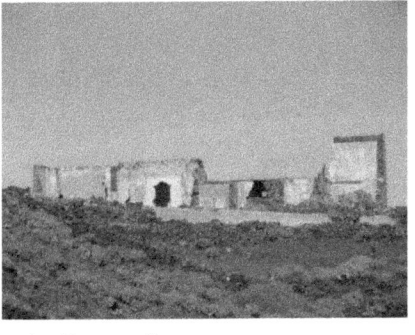 and back diversion will add 1-hour to the walk.

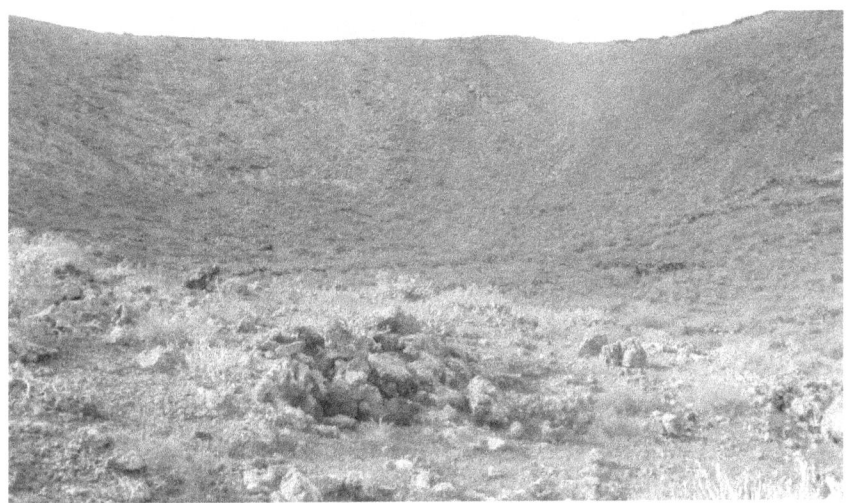

Notes

Charco Del Palo to Arrieta and Return

Walk North from Charco Del Palo, and stop when you reach Arrieta!

This is a 1½-hour, each-way, trainers, easy to find, level walk, along the beach/cliff giving remarkable views of the sea and energetic crashing waves.

Some walks take us over well-trodden paths where your heart-attack will see you discovered and revived in mere minutes. Others follow *the path less Travelled* (Frost,1920) so when you are eventually found it may be no more than your sun-bleached bones that remain to

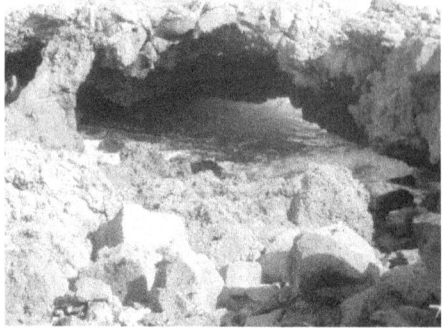

decorate the scenery . This one is pretty well walked; it's not remote, but a pleasantly quiet track. Not really bleached white bones territory.

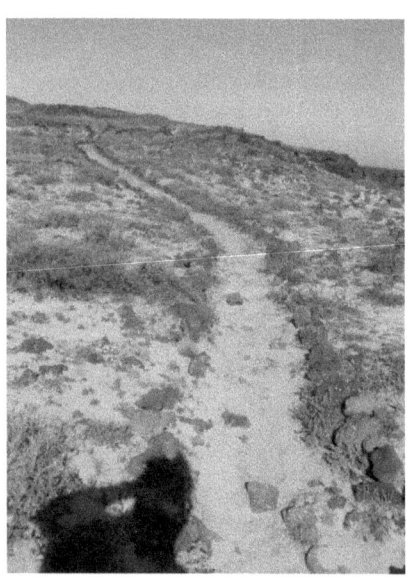

Parking in Charco is easy. Walk North and follow a path through the sand. There are many paths, so keep taking the options that most closely hug the sea.

We leave Charco heading north up the coast. The path is clear enough winding over sand and lava. The cliff is not high, but waves crashing on the lava are dramatic in places and if there's any wind expect spray.

Look out for stone designs and pods, everywhere. The spiral maze is popular on the island. Sometimes called a Celtic Maze, mazes have been found all over the world as far back as 3,500 BC. Purpose is unknown, but originally

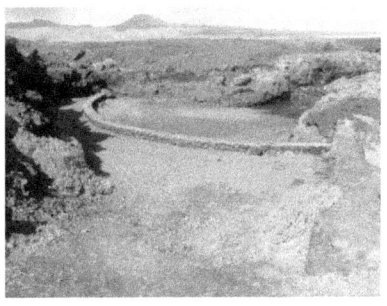

religious and more recently to walk them has been described as a form of meditation.

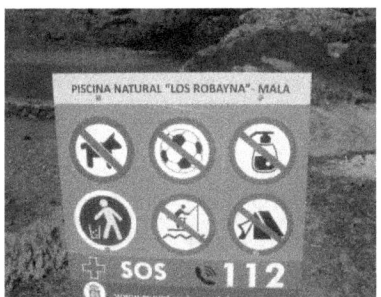

Anyway, we walk past a remote home, and the ubiquitous half-built house, and eventually, after nearly an hour reach a pleasant little man-made swimming bay. Mala's beach.

The usual Lanzarote *'Don't do anything at all'* sign applies. What the picture of a coffee jug is attempting to ban, I'm not entirely sure. 'No coffee!' seems a little harsh.

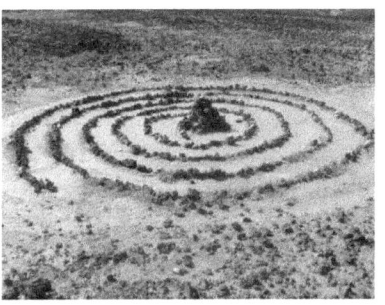

The path continues, without incident, just pleasant and easy strolling until we reach a beachside restaurant. This is a highly respected eatery, reasonably priced, so makes a fine lunch break on the beach. This is a good beach with golden sand favoured by campervans and tents. *(If we tell nobody, we could probably just return to Mala by the no:9 bus...)*

Refreshed, we retrace out steps and enjoy a post-perambulatory beer, this time in Reiners, pub. *None of us can explain why we keep torturing ourselves in this way and swear we'll never walk again, but we know we will.*

Las Calderas and Cocotaros

This is a 2-hour, trainers walk, not strenuous, with no risk of vertigo but some nice sea views.

Not remote. This is one of those walks that take us over well-trodden paths where your heart-attack will see you discovered and revived in mere minutes. Generally, we prefer *the path less travelled* where if you are ever found it will be no more than your bleached bones they discover decorating the scenery. Sadly, but this is none such.

We set out from the south end of Charco Del Palo, taking the jeep track up towards the mountain. We swing right and observe cairns on the hilltop to our right. Unlike many, these appear to be completely gratuitous, having no purpose at all. If we fancy an extra 2-minute climb, there is an excellent view back over Charco from these cairns. Ahead we soon see the paired mountains: Colorada and Mojon which give their named to Charco Del Palo roads.

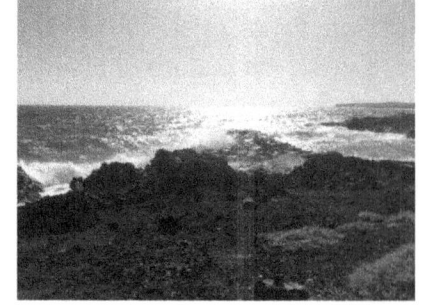

The track continues, heading towards a ruined farmhouse, which must have once been a glorious location overlooking the sea and the village but long since abandoned. Shortly before the final climb to that landmark we branch off to follow a track on the left. We might just trot up to the farmhouse for the view but if we do, we must walk back down to the fork.

Heading South, we skirt the foothills of Las Calderas, observing the farmhouses in the valley, each with its own means of channelling water into an al jibe. Presently, we see a large working quarry on the edge on Guatiza and just before this we take a fork heading West, towards the sea. We reach the coast and find a coastal path. If Cocotaros takes our interest, we can add a diversionary loop by trotting South on the costal path and seeing the 'town' with its unusual tidal swimming pool and then trotting back North.

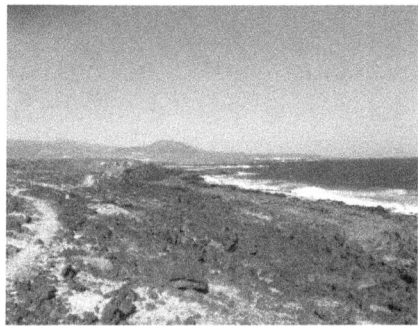

We want to head North along the costal path, passing close beside a nice farmhouse, where the path is made clear with a series of large arrows. Perhaps they don't want us straying into their garden.

We follow the path for perhaps ½-hour or so, pausing occasionally because the sea is pretty dramatic and the rocks impressive.

Eventually, the path takes us to a discontinued building from where it is good to ascend the mound of lava for the view and to admire the range of sunbathing pods. If we look down at the footings of the abandoned building, it would have been a fine location, but the layout of rooms is a serious puzzle, worthy of a little pondering.

> *It is interesting to study the stone pods giving wind protection to the sunbathers. These are frequently single layer of stones, one on another and look entirely fragile. The nature of the volcanic rock is such that it just locks together and lasts for ever. The pods on the beach are the same, of course.*

From there we recognise the track that we so unwisely followed two hours earlier and then we progress to the village and a bar for our usual post-perambulatory, cold beer. In comradely mood, we congratulate ourselves because, although we did allow ourselves to be seduced into (another) walk, at least it was only a relatively short one.

Mala Circle

First published as 🎵*Doing the Lambert walk*🎵 *on 'Alansblog',* 2016

This is a 3-hour, trainers, walk, moderately strenuous, with no risk of vertigo, in spite of a 400-m peak height. Fabulous views.

Take a compass, binoculars a map and your stick.

Quite remote, in places. Some walks take us over well-trodden paths where your heart-attack will see you discovered and revived in mere minutes. We love this one because it takes us on *the path less travelled* and when you are eventually found it will be no more than your bleached bones that remain to decorate the scenery.

This is a variant of a walk shown to us by Alan, last year. Alan's original walk is slightly gentler, but involves persuading a non-walker to drop you at the Chapel of the Snow by th golf ball from where we firstly 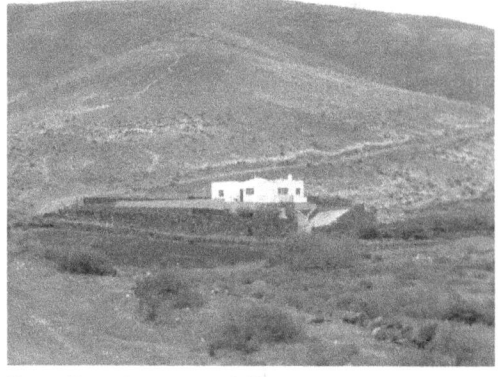 marvel at the view over Ilas Graciosa and Famara beach and then walk past The Golf Ball, down past The Dam and back to Charco del Palo, pausing only for a cold beer at The Arepera. Highly recommended if you have a kind driver and more so if you can persuade Alan to guide you because he'll give you snippets of history and agriculture that really do bring the scenery to life.

This walk suits us as we don't have a handy driver and want to walk up as well as down and on rougher tracks, not just farm roads.

We park by the church in Mala, which is at the North end of the town. If there were more than one car or there was a church service, then we'd park on the Mala main street.

We walk west down the road from the Church, crossing the LZ1 on a small bridge, and head gently uphill. We pass a farmhouse

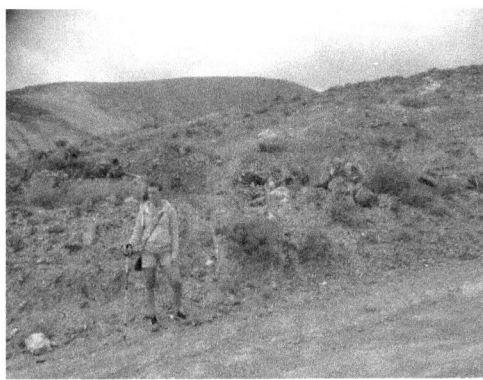

on our left, ignore a track to our left and then reach a white farmhouse on the right on a sharp right-hand bend. These houses are active farms. Both have serious solar arrays, suggesting that they may not be on the grid. There is a large water collection basin with a swimming pool type liner feeding a large Al jibe (Cistern) to supply a good array of fields, growing (Alan tells us) potato and watermelon.

To the Left of the track, opposite the white farmhouse on our right, there is a hard to discern path up the hill to the left of the road. Once we have scrambled up the initial bit this the path will become (fairly) clear.

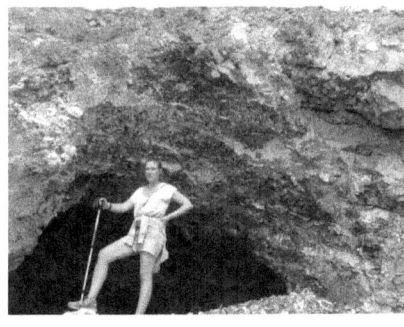

The track takes us up the hill always following the ridge looking down on cultivated valleys on either side. Along the way, beside the path we see little stone cairns. Some guidebooks say that these delineate ownership of land but others say they are used to define a path. We form the opinion that each is a memorial constructed for somebody who sadly died on one of Alan's more strenuous walks.

Perhaps a half-way up the ridge path there is a stone structure and a few cultivated terraces. Why just there is a puzzle worthy of a moment's pondering. To allow us to draw breath we feign interest in scenery and look behind us over Mala

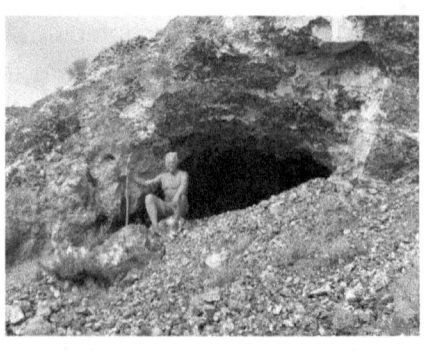

and Charco Del Palo. To the left we can see Arrieta, Punta Mujeres, Jamos Del Agua and beyond. Just to the left of the path near to this building a branch leads around to a hobbit hole/an extensive cave (a lava tube). Probably not entirely safe, but with a good torch at least we can look in from the cave mouth. The path to the cave is near the edge, but safe enough.

Continuing up the path is straightforward enough. When we near the top, it becomes considerably steeper but the path zig-zags and is in my opinion easy enough to find. In my companion's opinion, *"you're a total, ****wit, this isn't a path it's a watercourse, you're going to get us both killed….. and so on …and on…"* The reader must decide.

After zig-zagging for a bit it levels off at the top of the hill and you have easy walking for the rest of the journey. Shortly you find a dusty old stone wall to *step over.*

There are Classical Greek Myths where the souls of the dead cross a crumbling stone wall and descend to a dried up river bed and into oblivion. This wall exactly matches my image of that. It is a relief that we are crossing uphill into life, not downhill into death and oblivion.

Anyway, from here the path takes us up a dry watercourse, being very evident in places and invisible in others.

As we continue our gentle climbing, the golf ball hooves into view and this makes an excellent landmark. At every junction on our path we take the option that leads towards the golf ball.

This takes us onto a rough road and thence onto better roads until we pass a farmhouse distinguished by a rusty fence and drunken concrete gateposts.

We continue past that house and you reach a road junction with a larger house. Turn right, downhill, and we see a smart house on our right with what Alan calls *an unusual back garden*. (Massive lump of rock) From here, we follow the road to the left and the walk is a PoP *(No. You'll have to complete that acronym yourself)*

From there, we travel down the road, initially zig-zagging, and then straight, crossing the barranco (watercourse) by a ruined farmhouse in what must have been a lovely location. We proceed on down, passing a smart house/enclave, on the left, marvelling at the quite lush vegetation in places and eventually we see the dam on our left. It is possible to cross the dam,

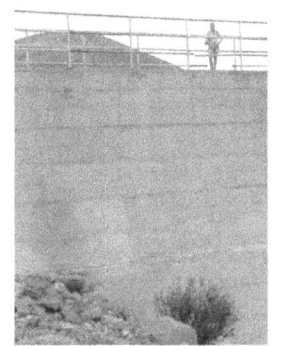 affording impressive views from the dam and the ridge beyond it unless for you, like me, vertigo prevails. There is always water in the dam but never very much. We're told that the dam has never actually worked, seemingly because the rock structure is too porous to hold water.

We cross back and head downhill. The road continues down, crossing another barranco, and loops nicely back to the white farmhouse where you so very unwisely decided to follow us and ascend by the path.

Returning to the car, we can drive home although, for us, tradition requires that we stop at The Arepera for very cold, post-perambulatory beer. That is a good time to berate ourselves for being so easily seduced into another torture walk.

Notes

Montana Tinamala, near Guatiza

This is a 1½ -hour, trainers, there & back walk, pretty strenuous in a health-giving way, with some risk of vertigo. Views of the coasts and lovely toy cars. Includesa rather unusual 'Egyptian' quarry.

Take a compass, binoculars a map and your stick. The path is a bit steep!

Quite remote, in places. Some of the route will take us over well-trodden paths where your heart-attack will see you discovered and revived in mere minutes. We love this one because most of it takes us on *the path less Travelled* (Frost,1920) and when you are eventually found it will be no

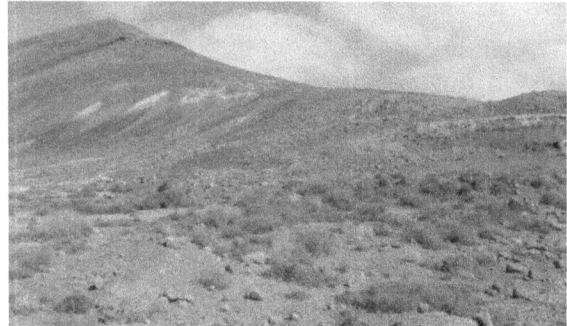

more than your bleached bones that remain to decorate the scenery.

Just off the LZ1 near Guatiza is a garage and shop with a large parking area on the dirt road behind.

Walk down the dirt road for a short way and look for a jeep path heading uphill on the left. Follow the track until you see a 'no entry' chain on the left. Pass through the 'no entry' and between two high cut walls to see a large space opening out in front of you.

This vaguely Egyptian looking structure was first a quarry but has

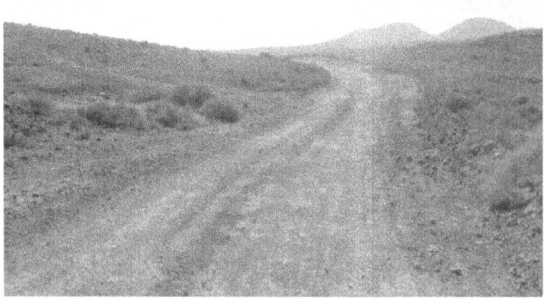

been many things since then, including a shooting range. Spot the bullet holes! What it the drain pipe for? Explore and marvel.

Leaving this first quarry, there is a track winding around the mountain and we soon see a second quarry looking far more Egyptian in style. In this one we can see that a huge al jibe has been fitted and we can see the chute where mountain run-off is

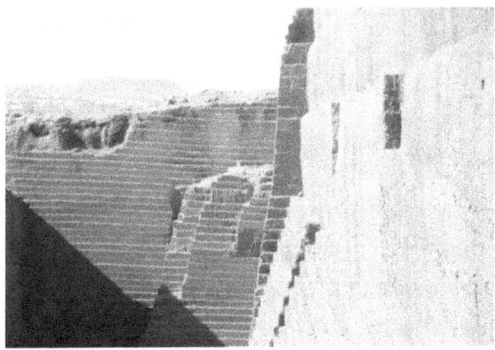

directed in. This small tank feeds into a very large one and the water can be directed through the drain pipe we saw earlier. That may have been used to drive a mill, or more likely to wet the blades of stone cutting machine. Having marvelled at this second hole, we return to the road and walk on it to circumnavigate the mountain giving us an ever changing vista.

Suddenly... Nothing happens! And then after a moment, it happens again!

OK. No it doesn't. But what is interesting is that the road goes nowhere. It stops after a while at a huge barranco and we realise that this is not so much a road as a device to channel water into the huge al jibe we explored a moment ago.

Returning to the quarries, we pass between them to the high side of the first one, keeping well way from the very precipitous and unguarded drop into the quarry. The views here frequently *'blow me away'* but not literally; try not to get distributed over the landscape by a gust of Lanzarote wind.

Passing the quarries, we can see a jeep track to the foot of the mountain, from where we climb the ridge all of the way to the cross at the top. It is frequently the easiest route up the mountain to find an arm like this and walk up the ridge. It always feels slightly like walking up one arm of an octopus to reach the head.

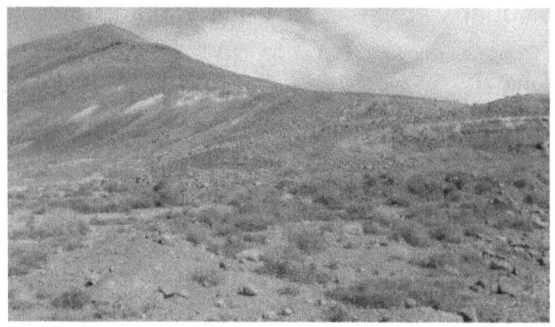 The route is quite steep and we gain height rapidly. Soon, looking to the left we see the ever-so-small LZ1, with its perfectly circular little roundabouts, the wee tunnel under the road and a tiny garage. Charming matchbox cars can be seen pulling into the perfectly detailed miniature filling station, each pretending to buy petrol. The effect is splendid; this is the toy car set that I always wanted.

Some mountains look intimidating and yet when you are climbing them they are no trouble at all. Others are the very opposite and this is one such. From the ground this is a kind and gentle mountain; butter would not melt in its mouth. However, when you are scrambling up, it may be necessary to look at your feet all of the way up, enjoy the peak and then walk gratefully down. If you experience vertigo, as I do, then 'Don't look down!' is very good advice. I gazed in delight at the toy car set until a part of my mind says, 'That's a long way down!' and I had to 'have-a-little-sit-down' until I felt belter. Then I had to make a change of underwear. Still, we only do it because we love it.

Anyway, the view from the top is fantastic and a map&compas will enable you to identify a good many features. That done and greatly enjoyed, we retrace our route to the wonderful sanctuary of the car with the Arepera in Mala only minutes away. The team there are poised, just waiting to serve us with ice-cold beer. Over that drink, always accompanied by complementary tapas, we should congratulate ourselves for taking only a relatively short walk; there are longer ones from Guatiza.

Guatiza Quarry

This is no more than ½ -hour, trainers, there & back walk, not strenuous in any health-giving way, with no risk of vertigo. Takes us to rather unusual 'Egyptian' quarry.

Not remote. The walk will take us over well-trodden paths where your heart-attack will see you discovered and revived in mere minutes. Really, we prefer walks that take us on *the path less Travelled* (Frost,1920) such that when you are eventually found it will be no more than your bleached bones that remain to decorate the scenery, but we can't win them all.

Just off the LZ1 near Guatiza is a garage and shop with a large parking area on the dirt road behind.We walk down the dirt road for a short way, admiring the high mountain on our Left and

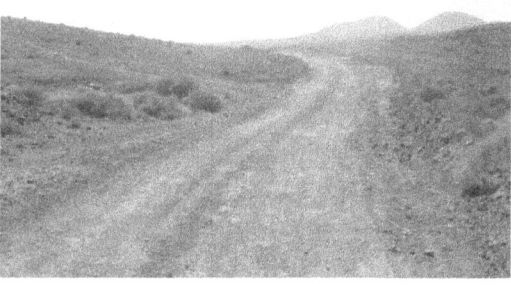

congratulating ourselves because we are not going to climb it.

After a few minutes we look for a jeep path heading gently uphill on the left.

Following the track we see a 'no entry' chain on the left. Passing through that 'no entry' portal and between two high cut walls we see a large space opening out in front of us.

This vaguely Egyptian looking structure was first a quarry but has been many things since then, including a shooting range. Spot the bullet holes! What it the drain pipe for? Explore and marvel.

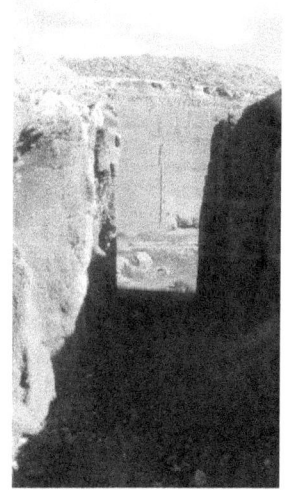

Leaving this first quarry, there is a track winding around the mountain and we soon see a second quarry looking far more Egyptian in style. In this one we can see that a huge al jibe has been fitted and we can see the chute by which mountain run-off is collected. This small tank feeds into a very large one and the water is directed through the drain pipe we saw earlier. That may have been used to drive a mill, (possibly to lubricate and cool cutting disks) but could just be an old water supply. Having marvelled at this second hole, we return to the road and walk it to circumnavigate the mountain giving us an ever changing vista.

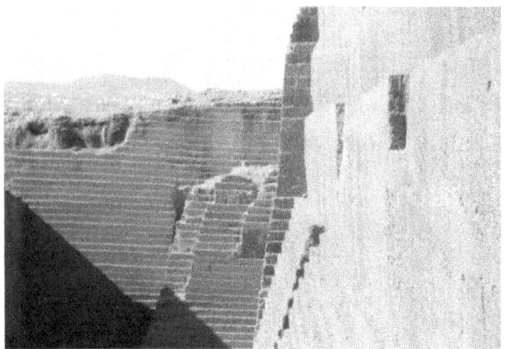

Suddenly... Nothing happens! And then after a moment...nothing happens, again!

OK. No it doesn't. But what is interesting is that the road goes nowhere. It suddenly stops at a huge barranco and we begin to think that this is not so much a road as a device to channel water into that huge al jibe which we explored a moment ago.

Returning to the quarries, we pass between them to the high side of the first one, keeping well way from the very precipitous and unguarded drop into the pit. The view frequently 'blows me away' but I try not to get distributed over the landscape by a gust of Lanzarote wind.

Passing the quarries, we can see a jeep track to the foot of the mountain and a path to the peak. Luckily for us, we are not going that way. We retrace our route to the wonderful sanctuary of the car with the Arepera in Mala only minutes away. Over a beer, always accompanied by complementary tapas, we should congratulate ourselves for taking only a relatively short walk when there are many far longer options in Guatiza.

Montana Teneje and fabulous barranco loop, Guatiza

This is a 2-hour, hard-soled, circular walk, only moderately strenuous in any health-giving way, with no risk of vertigo. It takes us up a spectacular barranco, returning over the mountain looking down over our path. The walk up does not feel strenuous at all, because the spectacle of the ravine is mesmerising.

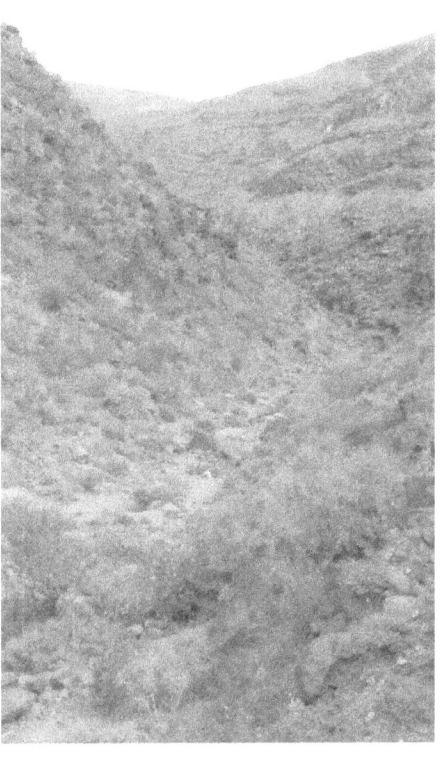

It's a little remote. Some walks take us over well-trodden paths where your heart-attack will see you discovered and revived in mere minutes This walk, however, takes us on *the path less Travelled* (Frost, 1920) such that when you are eventually found it will be no more than your bleached bones decorating the scenery.

Hard-soled boots and a stick would help.

Take the LZ1 to Guatiza take the small road to the West, crossing over the LZ1 bridge and park in the large area beside a large white building, (the graveyard)

Walk back down towards the bridge, but before reaching it take a path to the left. This is a typical Lanzarote elevated path on top of a wall, with the gulley on our Left and fields on our right. If there has been rain, there will be a good array of plants and

43

flowers including fig, nicotiana, rosemary, lavender, heather, and fennel, just as a starter. *Gardeners will be surprised by the nicotiana. This is not the decorative garden plant, nor yet the huge tobacco plant. This one grows into a shrubby, small tree. When it flowers, though, its ancestry becomes obvious.*

Periodically, the path fails and we walk in the gulley glad of our hard boots, but it always returns to us. Gradually, the climb steepens and presently we find ourselves stepping over larger rocks many in the form of a natural staircase. The rocks are smoothed by water, laced with sand and pecon. It is a testament to the vigour and abrasion of this abrasive 'soup' that these super-hard rocks have been smoothed off in a relatively short time.

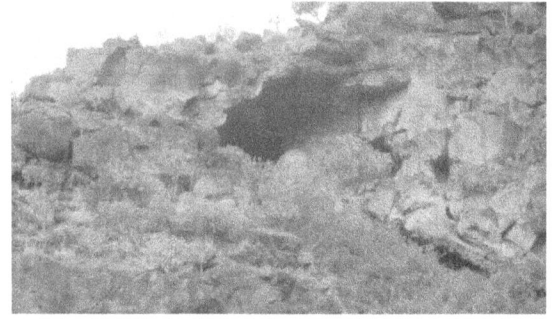

Eventually, the barranco becomes so steep that it cannot be further navigated. Here, for those who like such things, there is a *Geocache*. To our right, there is a nice group of hobbit holes set in the cliff and beyond that the crest of the hill, but not easily accessed by those without rope and good mountaineering skills. We take the far kinder path on the Left of the ravine, which gently brings us out onto the top of the gorge. Nearing the top, we again climb that dry stone wall over which (in myth anyway) dying souls pass and descend into death and oblivion. As ever, we are climbing up over, so we have no such depressing prospects.

The high ground is more barren but our path is (fairly) clear, guiding us back along the top of the cliff. To our right we can see and hear some of the windmills that give Lanzarote much of its power.

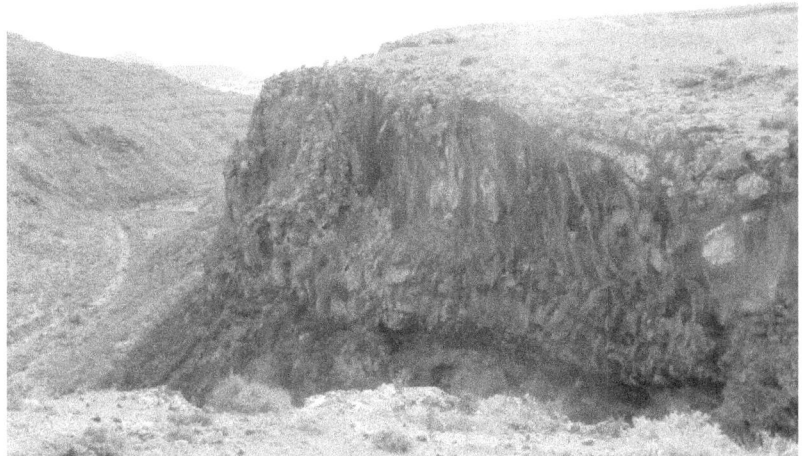

The view down into the barranco is, if it were possible, even more spectacular than it was viewing up from the barranco floor. The path is quite close to this very precipitous edge and I personally prefer to take one that is a little further inland. We gently ascend a little to reach the 265-Metre peak and then we begin a modest descent. Soon our parking place becomes visible in the distance so when the path occasionally fails us we have a clear landmark to guide us.

On reaching glorious sanctuary in the form of our transport, we could take comfort and post-perambulatory ale at the Arepera in Mala or, for adventure, park beside the Bulin's roadside bar in Guatiza for a bottle of Tropical. This frequently comes accompanied with a display of conjuring by the proprietor whose prestidigitation skills once provided him with a good living. Magic tricks at Bulin's Bar or iced-beer at Arepera, we must congratulate ourselves on selecting one of the shorter local walks, but how good would it have been if we had not even done that!

Notes

Montana De Guenia, Guatiza – for Los Ancianas

This is a 2-hour, trainers, circular walk, not strenuous in any health-giving way, with no risk of vertigo. It takes us halfway up the side of a fine Volcano, delivering fine views on a wide and secure path.

It's a little remote. Many walks take us over well-trodden paths where your heart-attack will see you discovered and revived in mere minutes. This walk will take us on *the path less Travelled*

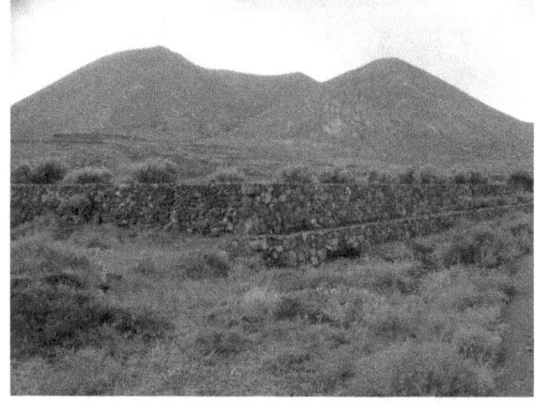

(Frost, 1920) such that when you are eventually found it will be no more than your bleached bones that decorate the scenery.

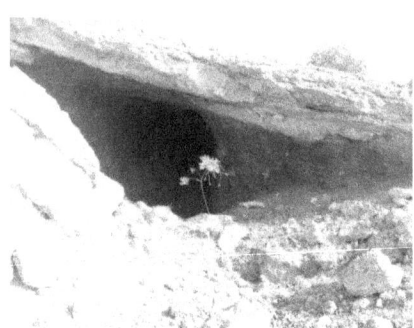

Take the LZ1 to Guatiza take the small road to the West, crossing over the LZ1 bridge and park in the large area beside the large white building, (the graveyard). Leave the car at the far end of the car park, near the Water Company building. We take the road to the right, North, loop sharply to the Left, crossing a watercourse and pass a farm. We ignore a jeep track on the left (our return road) and continue, firstly away from the mountain and then reaching a cross-road, take the Left turn to head back towards our hill. We continue around the mountain, watching the terrain changing, ignoring a turning to our Right until our road peters out to become a path. We pass a quarry

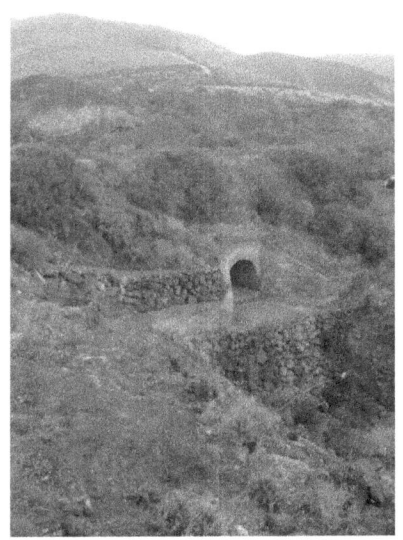 on the left and continue around, marvelling at all of the 'des-res' Hobbit Holes in the slope to our left. The path has a little downhill scramble and continues to our left on a wide track. We occasionally see a large pipe buried in the ground the purpose of which will become clear before long. The path is now about ½-way up the mountain but is wide and easy, maintaining a level trajectory. The views over Guatiza and the farmland are splendid and constantly changing as we progress around the mountain.

Soon we can see the car; far off for sure, but just to see it is so reassuring! We soon come to a water tower which explains the pipe we've been following. We cross over a shallow watercourse and to our Left we can see that we are nearly in the basin of the volcano. A short diversion up the watercourse and its attendant path puts us in the basin itself, which is well worth the extra effort. Standing and turning full circle gives the best effect of these basins.

Wowed by the volcano basin, we retrace our path down the watercourse to the jeep track and turn Left which takes us back to the road. It is a short step to the car and a shorter one to either Arepera at Mala or Bulins roadside bar in Guatiza for a bottle of Tropical. As we know, Bulin's beer frequently comes accompanied with a display of conjuring by the proprietor whose prestidigitation skills once provided him with a good living. Magic tricks or iced-beer at Arepera, we must congratulate ourselves on selecting one of the shorter and easier local walks, but how good would it have been if we had not even done that!

Montana De Guenia, Guatiza – for the intrepid

This is a 2-hour, trainers, circular walk, a little strenuous in any health-giving way, with great risk of vertigo and a degree of scrambling. It takes us up a barranco and over the peak of a

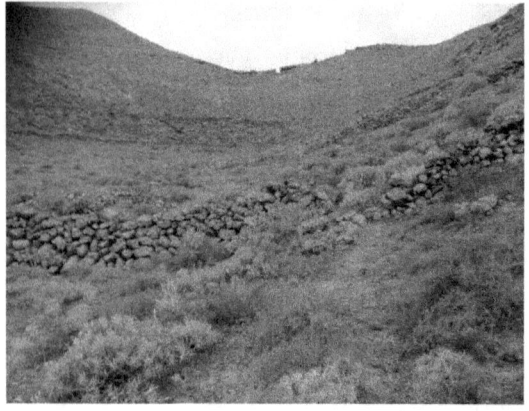

grand Volcano, delivering fine views on both sides if the mountain

It's a little remote. The walk will take us on *the path less Travelled* (Frost, 1920) such that when you are eventually found it will be no more than your bleached bones that remain to decorate the scenery.

Take the LZ1 to Guatiza take the small road to the West, crossing over the LZ1 bridge and park in the large area beside the large white building, (the graveyard). Leave the car at the far end of the car park, near the Water Company's building.

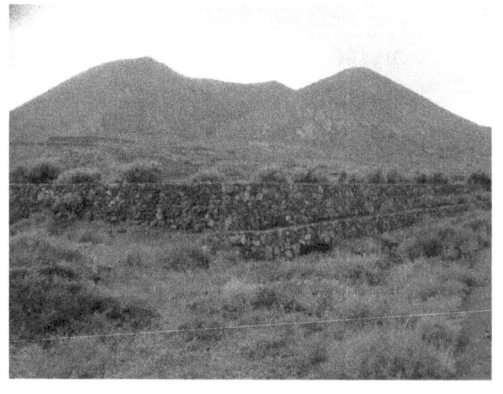

Walking on a path around the right-hand side of the Water building we will see a steep path upwards through a watercourse reaching a tar macadam road. We pass a farm and take a jeep track on the left. The track crosses a barranco and here we turn Right following the watercourse into the bowl of the volcano. Soon we see a path beside the barranco and following it takes us into the bowl of the volcano. Standing in the basin and turning full circle gives the best effect of these volcanoes. Wowed by the volcano basin, we press on upwards passing to the right of a field enclosure and see a path struggling to the volcano's ridge. Obtaining the ridge gives us spectacular views both East and West. If the wind was behind us on the ascent then the rocky ridge will give shelter. After enjoying this location, taking water and maybe food, we look for a route down the other side. This is not really a route; there are many *'sort of'* paths but no one in particular. Firm feet and a stick are needed because some of the stones are lose; we cautiously pick our way down. In another basin on the other side, we can see a *'sort of'* path winding around the lower

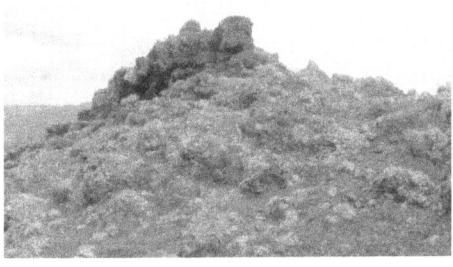

portion of the mountain. *(If you don't want any more 'sort of' paths, then it is possible to track to the right and join the farm road. This we would follow around the mountain before it shrinks to a path at a quarry and skirts the mountain all of the way back to the original tar macadam road.)*

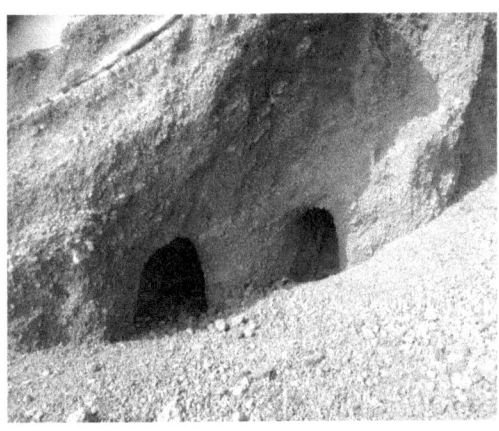

We, however, follow the *sort-of-path* around the mountain which climbs a little, coming and going, before finally taking us into a large quarry. Here we can see tracks where walkers have skittered down the stone to the path at the entrance of the quarry.

We pass another quarry on the left and continue around the mountain, marvelling at all of the 'des-res' Hobbit Holes in the slope to our left. The path has a little downwards scramble and continues to our left on a wide track. We occasionally see a large pipe buried in the ground the purpose of which we can't imagine. The path is now about ½-way up the mountain but is wide and easy, maintaining a level trajectory. The views over Guatiza and the farmland are splendid and constantly changing as we progress around the mountain.

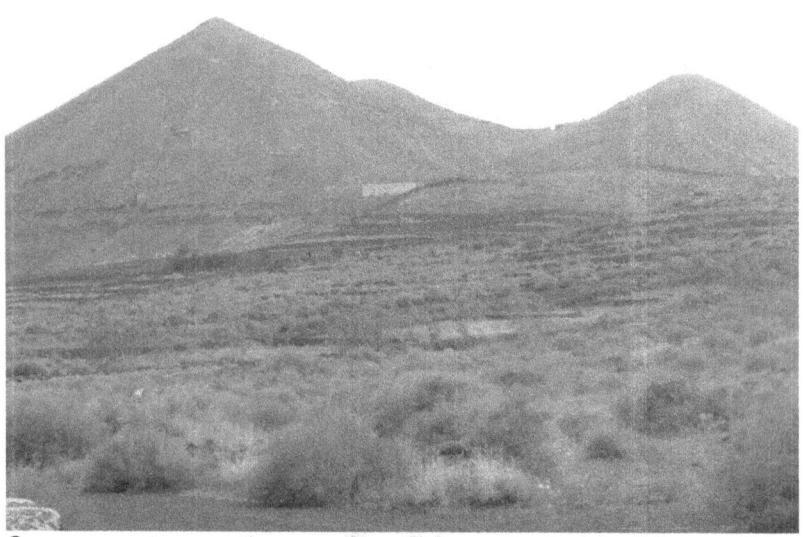

Soon we can see the car; far off for sure, but just to see it is a blessing! We soon come to a water tower which explains the pipe we've been following (OK I did know). We cross over a shallow watercourse and to our Left we can see that we are back at the basin of the volcano. It is a short step to the car and a shorter one to either Arepera at Mala or Bulins roadside bar in Guatiza for a bottle of Tropical. As we know, Bulin's beer frequently comes accompanied with a display of conjuring by the proprietor whose prestidigitation skills once provided him with a good living. Magic tricks or iced-beer at Arepera, we must congratulate ourselves on selecting one of the shorter and easier local walks, but how good would it have been if we had not even done that!

Bulins is a place to indulge our contemplation about which of us hates walking the most.

'Well of course walking for me is particularly difficult because one of my legs is shorter than the other'.

'One leg shorter than the other? That's nothing! One of mine is longer than the other and everyone knows that's much worse.'

Ha! A couple of mismatched legs is nothing; I've been walking for years with two arthritic hip joints'.

Only two arthritic joints? Luxury! I've had Arthritis, Rheumatism and Gout in every joint of my body for ninety-years and a broken ankle for the last ½-mile'.

'Arthritis, Rheumatism and Gout in every joint for ninety-years and a broken ankle. I long for such minor problems; you lot don't know what trouble is. I was born with no joints in my legs at all and had to ....'

Anyway, the beer is good and the road a constant source of interest. Consider what the bar must have been like before the LZ1 was built and this was the main road to the North.

Notes

Ye Montana Corona circuit

This is a 3-hour, trainers, walk, pretty strenuous in a health-giving way, with minimal risk of vertigo. Views of the East and West coasts. Great viewing into the volcano basin, far below.

Take a compass, binoculars a map and your stick. The path is not entirely trustworthy!

Quite remote, in places. Some of the route will take us over well-trodden paths where your heart-attack will see you discovered and revived in mere minutes. We love this one because much of it takes us on *the path less Travelled* (Frost,1920) such that when you are eventually found it will be no more than your bleached bones that remain to decorate the scenery.

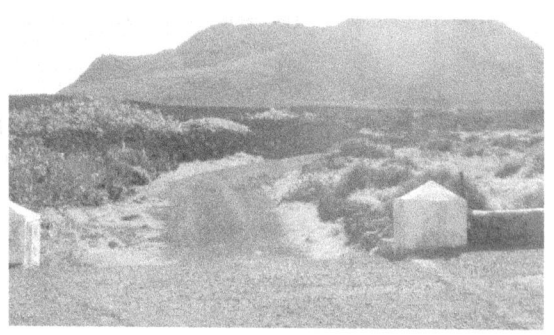

The entrance to the track is between the Church and the Sociodad in Ye High Street. We can usually park at the entrance to the track but should there be no spaces left, then there are spaces aplenty by the church.

This road rolls through good cultivation mostly Grape Vines, interspersed with Fig and Olive and the occasional majestic Lanzarote Palm.

> *Many years ago, somebody introduced these palms to the island and was pleased to see them thrive. However, I will never forgive him for not favouring a variety that actually produces edible dates. There is nothing like a date straight from the tree, but the Lanzarote date is quite inedible. It*

does, however, germinate easily so you might take a handful home.

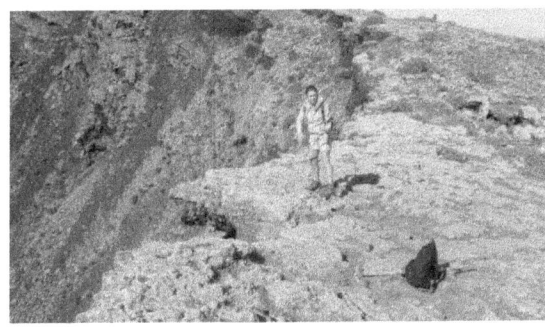

Anyway, the road abruptly ends and a path continues between two cairns up and up until it, too, fails and a steep scramble ensues. We scramble on until we broach a wall. This is another of those dry walls reminiscent of the mythical barrier over which the soul passes in death to progress down to a dry river and oblivion. I only mention this as we are passing over it upwards into life. Were we heading down towards death and oblivion I would not have brought it up.

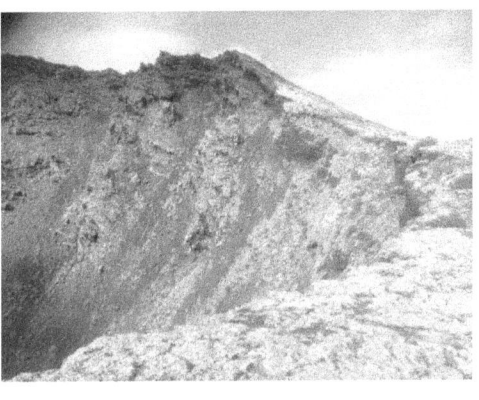

Anyway, the view into the mountain is suddenly upon us and it takes your breath! We view high peaks to Left and Right and straight ahead there is a dramatic drop to the basin of the volcano.

It is possible to walk down into the basin; there is a track. However, it is a fair old challenge so up to you. *I don't want to be called a ***wit (again).*

It is also possible to climb the two peaks, but this is not an entirely safe climb if there is any wind at all it is not recommended (nor is it particularly worth it).

From here, we walk down a track on our Left, following a stone wall, through cactus fields.

The track is on the Left-hand side of the wall, but eventually we need to be on the Right; we'll need to cross, but you can choose where. The problem is that since our Mr Lambert first developed the walk a fence has been added to the wall, probably to stop goats. The first and clearest option (which I will call, *'Option 1'*) is to descend right into the corner of the wire fence, where it is clear from minor damage that people cross over the fence at their right hand. From here, slightly downhill to our left, there is a high path, built on the top of a wall in the Lanzarotean way. This continues, to become a standard, fairly clear path that winds right around the mountain.

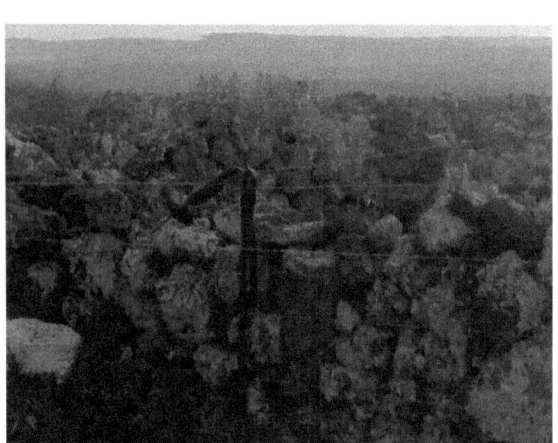

Alternatively (and this I will call, *'Option 2'*) higher up there is an area where the fence is lowered and rudimentary steps are in place. From here a faint, but definite path exists downhill angling away from the wall until it meets up at right-angles with the path-proper that curls around the mountain as in option 1.

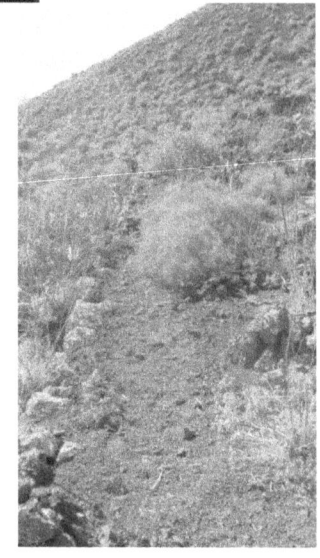

What I am going to call, *'Option 3'* is to cross the wall before even the fence starts, where the stone has fallen away. We descend, hugging the wall until reaching one of the paths described in option 1 or option 2.

All options work, the reader decides.

From here the path winds horizontally around the mountain through pecon and cinders and occasional farmed areas under this dramatic mountain peak. There are quite dramatic views, because we are still very high, but vertigo does not seem to strike. We walk on around the mountain with a constantly shifting vista until finally we reach a quarry and a scramble down to the road.

On reaching the cinder road and having eaten, imbibed and removed pecon from our shoes, we turn right and head South-West on the track until on our Right we reach a large al jibe with an enormous cement water collection surface. This is visible from many miles away on the island. Visiting it may answer a question for you, if you've been wondering what it was, as I had done for years.

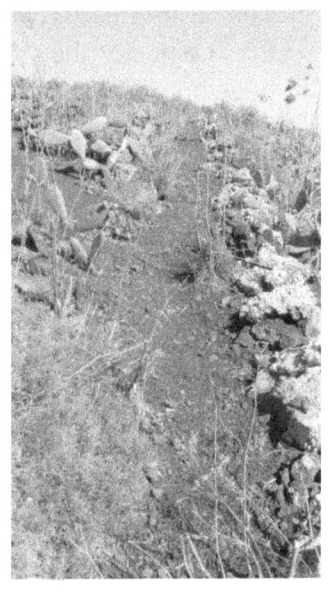

We hop up onto the collection concrete and traverse it until we reach the top left corner and set off over the ground. From here the path is unreliable and the more you seek it, the more it will hide, but we don't mind because we work on the basis that we can just follow the contour line around the mountain. So - neither uphill nor downhill. There is a jeep track near the al jibe but that goes too high up the slope and suddenly ends; don't go that way. Rather, follow the faint foot paths around the mountain. Here Hiawatha might be a useful companion.

As we round the mountain we start to see terraced fields and then a strong black stone wall looms out ahead. This is clear because the terrace walls are white stone. *(Actually they're black stone, but covered with white lichen.)*

Making a bee-line for the straight black wall miraculously puts us onto a strong footpath and it is a puzzle how we missed it until now. The answer is that it 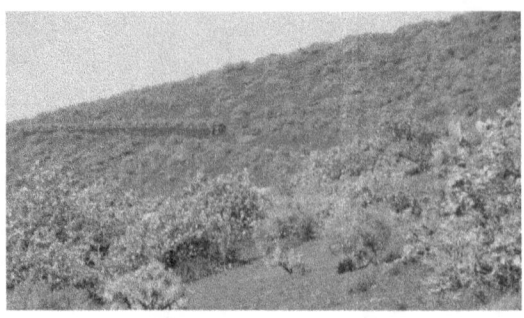 is one of those Lanzarote *Hogwart's paths*; it comes and goes at will and especially so if sudden absence will result in inconvenience.

We've got the path now and can follow it easily until we reach a pecon quarry and scramble down a track to the tar macadam road.

This is the LZ201 which we cross near a palm tree and follow the track to the West. We pass the ubiquitous half-built development on our Left, *'The cliffs de Guinate'*, and reach a white house on our right. Opposite the white house there is a Jeep track on our left. We follow that track all of the way to the edge of the cliff.

Disturbingly close to this 400-metre high sheer-drop cliff is the cliff path. From there, the view is *Really-Quite-Impressive*. Follow the path around to the right (North), for about ½-hour.

This is not a place to stumble. We *Walk – stop – look; walk - stop – gaze; walk - stop – stare; walk - stop – gape; walk - stop – gawk;* etc until we are completely out of synonyms.

On this path when walking, we look at our feet; when admiring the view we *stand dead still!!*

If you have vertigo, of if there is any wind, then you might use a second path which is some little way further from this most precipitous of cliffs.

At the end of this section, we reach a stone wall and step over it to see a path heading down to the left into a green valley. We go down, heading towards a remote farm house on the cliff, but before reaching it we branch sharply to the right, heading for another jeep track in the valley. We cross a small (dry) stream over a tiny clapper bridge and stop awhile to admire the terraced hills that almost completely surround us. We use the tar macadam track to return to the LZ201. This takes us past a smart aloe vera field; very impressive when they are in flower in the autumn.

Reaching the road we walk Left, into Ye and back to the blessed safety of our car.

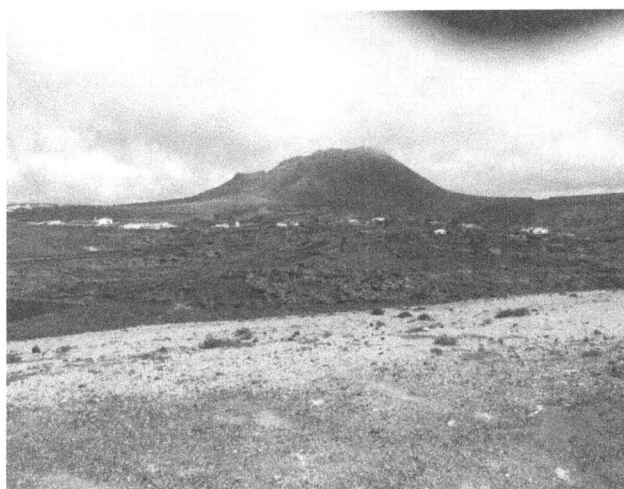

Returning to the car, we can drive 100-yards to the Sociodad for our usual post-perambulatory, cold beer. From there we ask ourselves how we allowed ourselves to be seduced into (another) walk, and not altogether a short one, either.

Notes

Ye Quemada and Corona circuit

This is a 3-hour, trainers, walk, pretty strenuous in a health-giving way, with small risk of vertigo. Pleasant views of two volcanoes and into the basin, far below, of one.

Popular in part, but remote in places. Where, taking *the path less Travelled* we will only be found as sun-bleached bones.

Take a compass, binoculars a map and your stick.

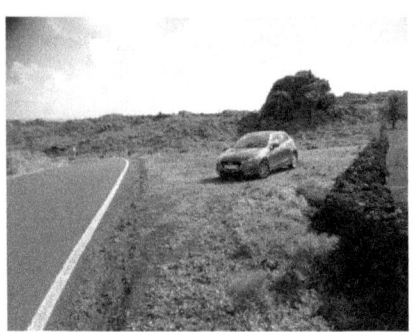

We can park on the Road from Orzola to Ye, before it reaches the LZ201, a little North (downhill) from Casa La Brena. There is a good parking area on the bend.

Head up the hill, using the roadside walkway which constitutes part of the Orzola to Playa Blanca island route. (A real marathon – at best three days.)

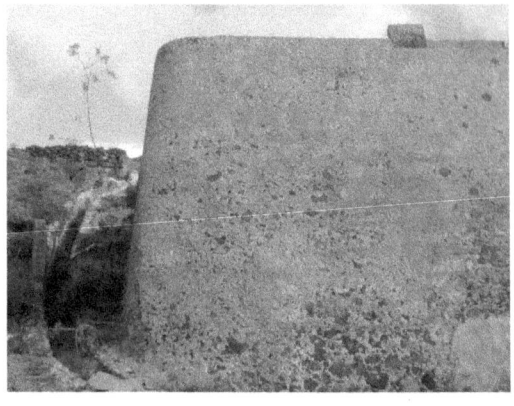

We soon turn Right up a farm cinder track skirting and climbing La Quemada through some limited cultivation and with a splendid valley view to our right. We roach the mountain pass after 20-mins and descending find an imposing structure, labelled RRNOBE, presumably built in 1949.

This is an intriguing building, which requires 10-mins exploration. Climbing to the top is facilitated by two steps in the wall. Once you've worked it all out, *(it's a mill)* we continue down the path, through rich cultivation across a verdant basin before climbing back up to reach the road. Cross straight over to join the Ye high street. On our Left we pass the Sociodad, *(too soon for a beer?)* then we ignore the first road on the left and ditto the first path before taking the main track left towards the mountain, far above.

This road rolls through good cultivation mostly Grape Vines, interspersed with Fig and Olive. The road abruptly ends and a path continues between two cairns up and up until it, too, fails and a steep scramble ensues. We scramble on until we broach a wall. This is another of those dry walls reminiscent of the mythical barrier over which the soul passes on death to progress down to a dry

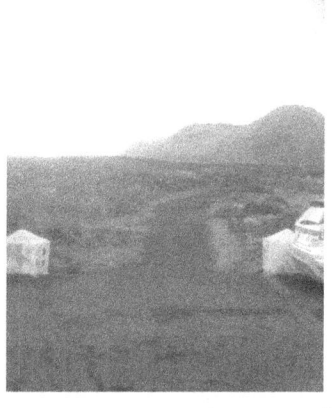

river and oblivion. I only mention this as we are passing over it upwards into life. Were we heading down towards death and oblivion I would not have mentioned it.

Anyway, the view into the

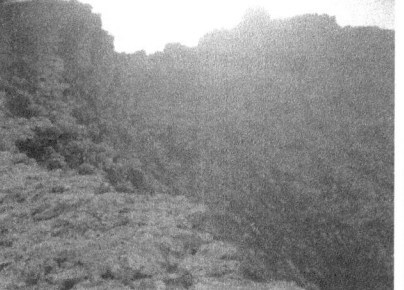

mountain is suddenly upon us and takes your breath!

It is possible to walk down into the basin; there is a

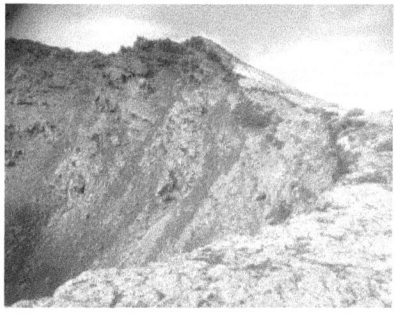

track. However, it is a challenge so make your own decision. I don't want to be called a ***wit (again).

From here, we walk down a sort of track on our Left, following a wall, through cactus fields.

The track is on our (Left) side of the wall, but eventually we need to be on the Right. We'll need to cross, but you can choose where. The problem is that since Mr Lambert first developed the walk a fence has been added to the wall, probably to stop goats. The first and clearest option (option 1) is to descend right into the fence corner, where it is clear that people cross the fence. From here, slightly downhill to our left, there is a high path, built on the top of a wall in the Lanzarotean way. This continues to become a standard, fairly clear Path that winds right around the mountain.

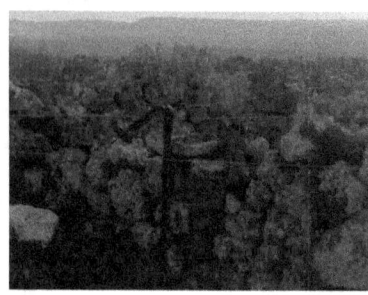 Alternatively (Option 2) higher up there is an area where the fence is lowered and rudimentary steps are in place (below). From here a faint, but definite path exists downward until it meets up at right-angles with the path that curls around the mountain as in option 1.

Option 3 is to cross the wall before the fence starts, where the stone has fallen away. We descend, hugging the wall until reaching one of the paths either in option 1 or option 2.

All options work, the reader decides.

From here the path winds horizontally around the mountain through pecon and cinders. There are quite dramatic views, because we are still high, but vertigo does not seem to strike. We walk on around the mountain with a constantly shifting vista until finally we reach a quarry and a scramble down to the road. Turning Left, we follow the cinder track, again part of the Orzola to Playa Blanca path, as signs periodically tell us. This road emerges onto the LZ201, under a fine chateau and we turn Left to use the road for a very short stretch.

Soon we leave the LZ201, taking a track on the right, signed as the Orzola to Playa Blanca path. In fact, we go straight on, when the main road (LZ201) swings to the left.

This track continues down through good cultivation and charming countryside, until returning to the original tar macadam road near where we so foolishly left our car. We turn Left and walk for just ten minutes and are delighted to find our car where we left it in pursuance of this quixotic and quite ill-advised quest.

The nearest post-perambulatory cold beer is the Ye Sociodad, but we could probably practice delayed gratification and drive for a further ten-minutes to get a super-cold beer from the Arepera in Mala. Here, we can hold a strict post-mortem deciding just whose fault it is that we went for a walk this time.

Notes

The best views on the island – Guatifay

(There are a lot of contestants for that title, but we stand by our judgement)

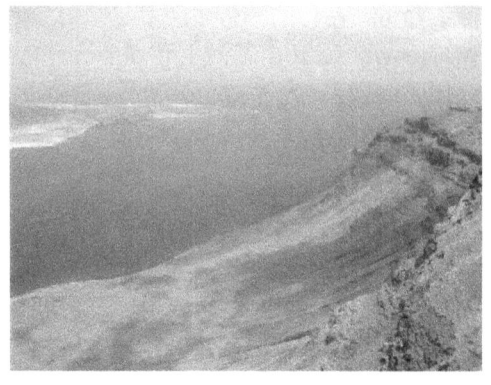

This is a 1-hour, trainers walk, not strenuous, with only minimal risk of vertigo, in spite of a 400-m cliff height. Quite Fabulous Views. Best sighting of Isla Graciosa on the island! Preferably no wind and good visibility.

Take a compass, binoculars and a map.

Not remote. Some walks take us over well-trodden paths where your heart-attack will see you discovered and revived in mere minutes. We prefer those that take us on *the path less Travelled* and when you are eventually found it will be no more than your bleached bones that remain to decorate the scenery. However, this is none such.

Ok, so this is a gentle and short walk of only an hour or so, but we'd better add on however long we want give to standing and being astounded by what we see. *(The view is quite good!)*

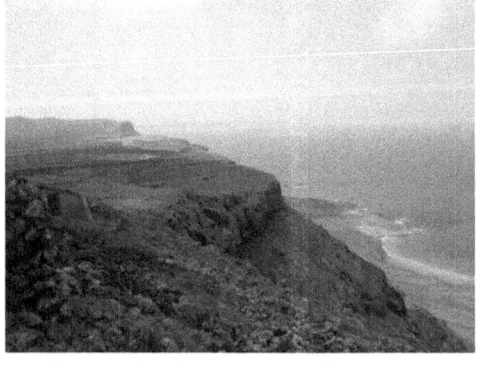

Take the LZ201, North, from Maguez passing the turning on the left for the Guinate Tropical Park. Shortly after that we reach another turning on the left, sporting a fine palm tree, opposite a quarry, signed Camino De Guatifay.

Park near the tree and set off up the road to the West. We pass the ubiquitous half-built development on our left, *'The cliffs de Guinate'*, and reach a white house on our right. Opposite the house there is a Jeep track on our left. We follow that track all of the way to the edge of the cliff.

Disturbingly close to this 400-metre high cliff is the cliff path. From there, the view is *Really-Quite-Impressive*. Follow the path around to the right (North), for about ½-hour.

This is not a place to stumble. Walk – stop – look; walk - stop – gaze; walk - stop – stare; walk - stop – gape; walk - stop – gawk; etc until we are completely out of synonyms.

> *On this path when walking, we look at feet; when admiring we stand dead still!*

At the end of this section, we reach a stone wall and step over it to see a path winding down to the left into a green valley. We go down, heading towards a remote house on the cliff, but before reaching it we branch sharply to the right, heading for another jeep track at the bottom of the slope. We cross a small (dry) stream on a tiny clapper bridge and use the tarmac road to return to the LZ201. This takes us past a smart aloe vera field which can be pretty impressive in autumn, when they are in flower.

Reaching the road we walk Right, uphill, puffing a little for the good of our health, back to the car. This little section is not quite the dull trudge over tarmac that it might be as we are pretty impressed by the farm in the valley to our left. Another sight we'd never see from the car.

Returning to the car, we need to drive to find a bar for our usual post-perambulatory, cold beer. From there we congratulate ourselves because, although we did allow ourselves to be seduced into (another) walk, at least it was only a short one.

Notes

Costa Teguise to Los Cocoteros

This is 2-hours each-way, level, trainers walk, easy to find, with jolly good views of the white sea foam on the mad, black shapes of rock. Suitable for a windy day.

Take your stick for the rocky areas.

Quite remote, in places. Some walks take us over well-trodden paths where your heart-attack will see you discovered and revived in mere minutes. We love this one because it takes us on *the path less travelled* (Frost,1920) and when you 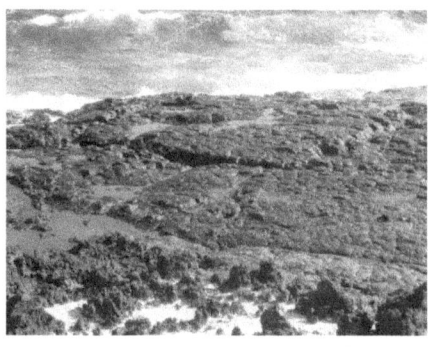 are eventually found it will be no more than your bleached bones remaining to decorate the scenery.

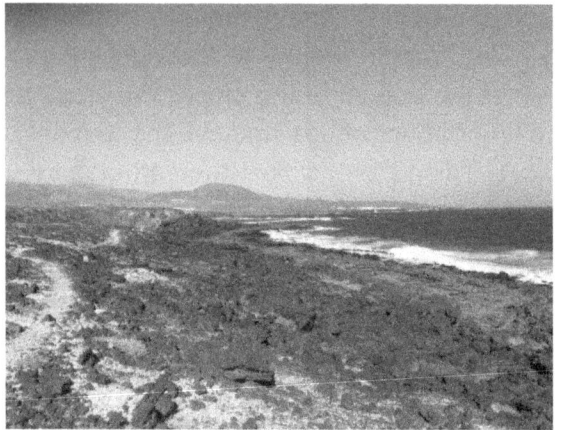

This walk is a matter of following the trail and, beyond recommending it very highly, there is little to explain. The walk is great with a little wind, when we get occasional light spray and watch white waves on magical lava shapes. There are tunnels, bridges and towers in the rocks. In places rock pools erupt into little geysers when waves crash into underwater lava tunnels and water is forced up into the pool.

The full journey takes at least 2-hours each way, but there is little to see in Cocoteros, beyond active salt pans and a quixotic

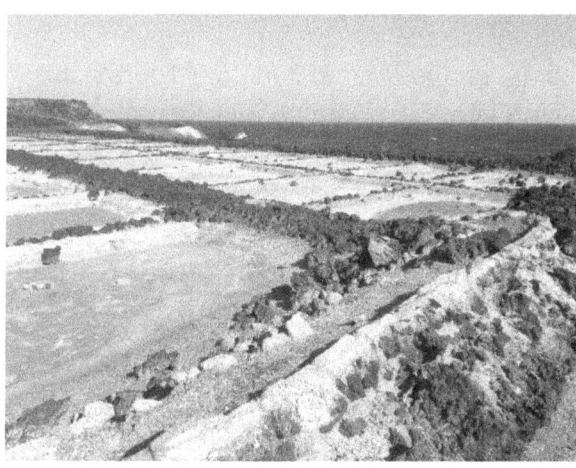 tidal pool; it is the sea front that is so magical. The walk can be set to any length we desire. For a 2-hour, walk for 1-hour and make an about turn. The experience well rewards the effort.

Leave Punta Corvina, heading North along one of the several available paths. There are multiple paths over much of this coast and the best effect is usually to select the one nearest the sea. Occasionally we find it is a dead-end and have to retrace our steps, but this is rare. In many places the track is marked by 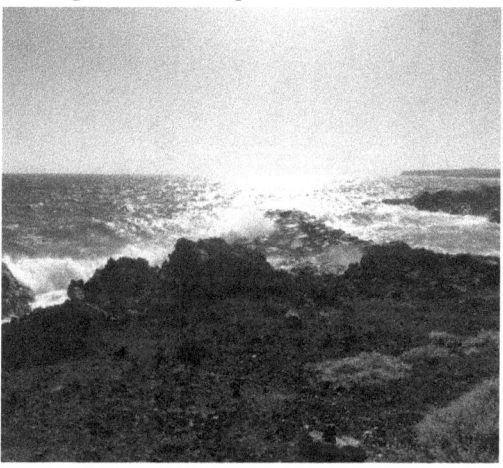 small bollards that actually define the coast line but also serve to pick out the cliff path.

Notes

Montana Corona, Costa Teguise

This is a 2-hour, circular, trainers walk, mostly easy to find, with one steep and tricky hill section that'll give you vertigo, followed by restful descents, and jolly good it is, too! There's that risk of vertigo, walking on the 230-m corona, but the path is wide and affords fine views. If you don't fancy the scary climb or if it is too windy, give some thought to the neighbouring and appositely named Montana de Saga.

Not suitable for a windy day!

Take a compass, binoculars a map and your stick.

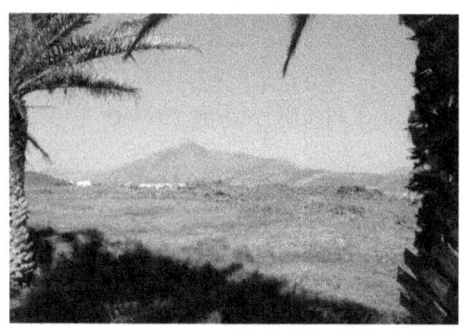

Quite remote, in places. Some walks take us over well-trodden paths where your heart-attack will see you discovered and revived in mere minutes. We love this one because it takes us on *the path less travelled* (Frost, 1920) and when you are eventually found it will be no more than your bleached bones remaining to decorate the scenery.

We park on the new, un-numbered road that runs from the folly by the LZ1 to Costa Teguise and we park by the mountain, ¼-mile before the T junction.

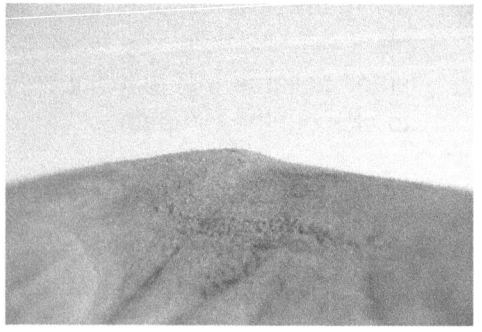

There is a barranco running up the mountain ahead of us and some people choose to scramble up in the comfort of this ravine, and that is fine to do.

However, we will look to the Left (NW) of the ravine and see that there is a path, which we will employ.

This starts easily enough, but like many mountain paths, it gets steeper and less distinct as we ascend. *"You're a total, ****wit, this isn't a path it's a watercourse, you're going to get us both killed..... and so on ...and on..."* However, a general, careful progress upwards with or without a path eventually gets us to the post at the peak. From here, the view over the sea, Costa

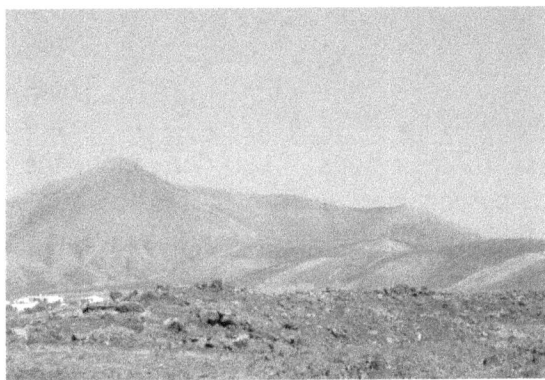

Teguise and Arrecife are pretty impressive. The oddly green area to the South West is the golf course.

From here it is fairly easy to follow the corona clockwise around the mountain stopping frequently to note the changing views. At the end of the corona there is a gentle(ish) path down to the plain.

Reaching a sort of crossroad, we turn Right and the path takes us into the volcano's basin. We enjoy this for a bit and continue around the mountain. We pass straight over another (sort of) cross road and eventually this path returns us, thankfully, to our start point.

We have climbed the mountain, circumnavigated it at the top and then reversed our circular patrol at the mountain base. *We must be mad!*

Reaching to the car allows us to return to base and seek out our usual post-perambulatory, cold beer and argue about whose fault it was, this time, that we decided to climb a mountain. *Never again!*

Montana de Saga – peak, Costa Teguise

This is a 1-hour, up-and-back, trainers walk, easy to find, with

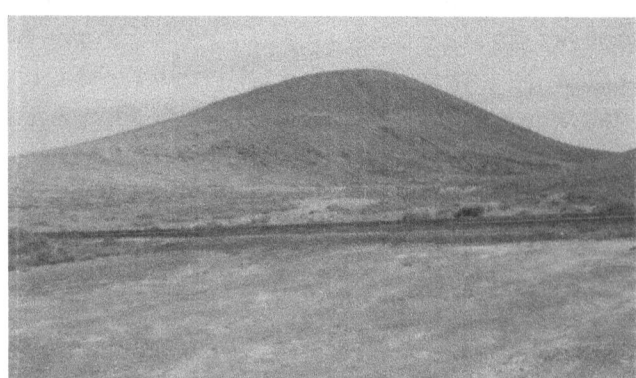

one simple but steep hill section, followed by brilliant views and restful descents. There's no real risk of vertigo, in spite of a 225-m peak. If you don't fancy the scary climb of Montana corona, next door, or if it is too windy, give some thought to this appositely named Montana de Saga.

Not too bad even on a windy day!

Quite remote, in places. Some walks take us over well-trodden paths where your heart-attack will see you discovered and revived in mere minutes. We love this one because it takes us on *the path less travelled* (Frost,1920) and when you are eventually found it will be no more than your bleached bones that remain to decorate the scenery.

Take a compass, binoculars a map and your stick.

From the LZ1, take the un-numbered road under Manrique's Gatehouse, towards Costa Teguise. Pass over a bridge, through No-overtaking signposts and there is ample parking on the Right. From Costa Teguise, walk or drive out towards the LZ1, NW, until you nearly reach the No-overtaking signs.

The two mountains: Corona and Saga are to the North-East of the road. Corona is a more tricky ascent, but both are the same height and give fine views.

The parking spot is beside a picturesque quarry or it's just possibly land sculptured by wind and rain. This is fascinating and merits a few 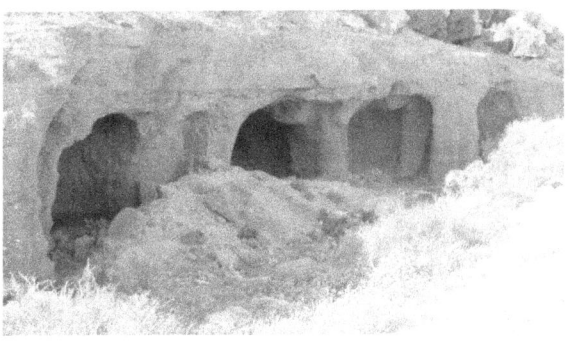 minutes' exploration. There are delightful natural sculptures and a good range of 'Hobbit Holes' any one of which would rent out for £50/night in the UK.

That done, we head towards the 'left-hand' mountain and see a clear track ascending the slope to the peak.

On the ascent, we pass a number of small barrancos (gulleys) taking water off the mountain. In several places it is interesting to see where these have been diverted and if we track them down we can see a verdant farm collecting all of that mountain water run-off.

Plodding on towards the peak, the path becomes steeper and looser, so our stick makes a welcome third point of contact with the ground.

The peak is worth a wonder-around and affords a dramatic view of part of Costa Teguise, Los Cocotaros and Charco Del Palo, on the coast; and Teseguite, El Mojon and Guatiza to our North. Montana Tinamala, near Guatiza looks inviting; a climb for another day.

It is possible to descend by either of the volcano's 'arms' and thereby make the walk a circular one but it is a tricky descent, and probably not worth the difficulty afforded.

The car is visible from the peak, so the descent is self-evident. Eventually, the slope levels out and it is a pleasant stroll back to the car and the wonderful security of its steel boxiness.

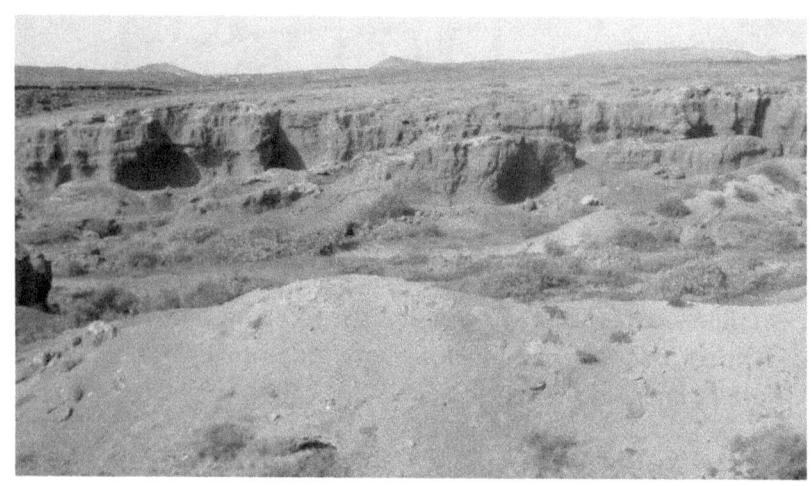

We repair to Mala and the Arepera for a post-perambulatory cold beer and (no for the first time) a *'Why do we do this?'* conversation.

Notes.

Montana de Saga circuit, Costa Teguise

This is a 1½ -hour, circular, hard-soled shoes walk, mostly easy to find, and jolly good it is, too! If you don't fancy the scary climb to the mountain peaks, or if it is too windy, this appositely named Montana de Saga ground level circuit is really enjoyable. Circumnavigating a volcano at near-ground level gives a view that is constantly changing from coastal villages, to mountains and inland towns. Each face of the volcano is unique, so the terrain is constantly changing and always

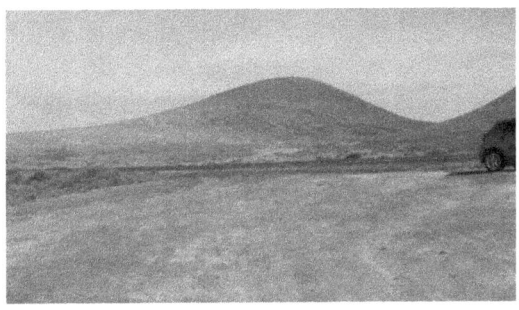

interesting. As we travel we encounter remarkable ravines and gulleys and begin to realize just how much water runs off these mountains.

Perfect for a windy day!

Take a compass, binoculars and a map.

From the LZ1, take the un-numbered road under Manrique's Gatehouse, towards Costa Teguise. Pass over a bridge, through No-overtaking signposts and there is ample parking on the Right. From Costa Teguise, walk or drive out towards the LZ1, NW, until you nearly reach the No-overtaking signs.

The two mountains: Corona and Saga are to the North-East of the road. Corona is a more tricky ascent, but both are the

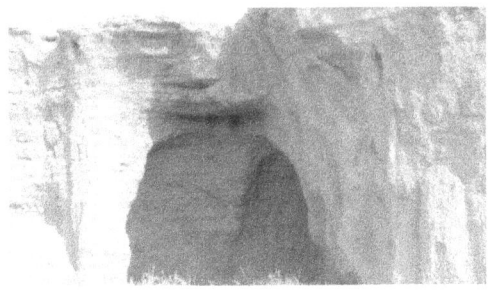

same height and afford us fine views.

The parking spot is beside a picturesque quarry or it has just possibly been sculptured by wind and rain. This is fascinating and merits a few minutes' exploration. There are delightful natural sculptures and a good range of 'Hobbit Holes' any one of which would rent out for £50/night in the UK.

That done, we take a cycle path that ascends the cleavage between our two mountains. As the path obtains its high point, the sea comes into view. Soon it is good to strike off the path to our Left and travel cross-country keeping the mountain on our left elbow. There is no path for us here. *(Actually, there is a path, but more of that later.)* Always keeping the mountain on our left elbow we encounter ravines and circumnavigate deep gulleys and with a little imagination can picture the scene during a decent rain storm!

> *Slowly, we travel around the mountain, rappelling down into galleys and grapple hooking ourselves out, or assembling small bailey bridges (or.. or.. or we can just go around them) until…*

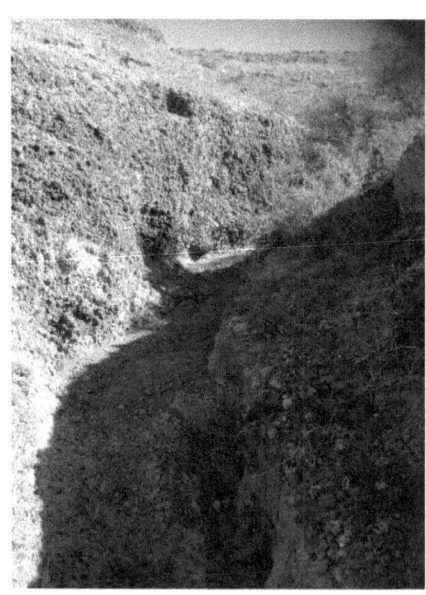

About ½-way around we are in a muddy basin and there is a dried up stream bed running our way. It is good to walk up the stream bed; it is easier than negotiating rocks and as we progress the walls become higher and the ravine deeper. Before long we can barely see out of our gulley. The gulley forks and divides and we always take the right-hand option, away from the mountain, as all of the gulleys will eventually go up the mountain.

We climb out of our last gulley and suddenly we spot a path. Climbing on to it we see that is even and clearly visible as far as the eye can see in both directions. Why was this not recommended by Lambert and Wheeler? This is one of Lanzarote's renowned Hogwart's paths that appear and disappear at will. I personally think that they do so to inconvenience walkers.

> Jerome K Jerome says of kettles, 'one must pretend to take no notice of it, if you want it to boil. It is a good plan, too, to talk loudly about how you don't need tea and will not drink any of it and would really prefer lemonade.'
>
> I find the same works for some paths. If I say 'look for path A or take track B' you will not find either in a month of weekends. If we pretend not to care about paths at all, then one will pop up in no time. Just until it thinks you are beginning to like following it and then it will instantly vanish. I tried a good trick on this one. I turned and followed it backwards and there it was as clear as day. Happy to be followed as long as it thought it was leading me in the wrong direction. Before long it smelled a rat and realized that I was liking following it and then 'Poof!' it was gone.
>
> So, suddenly we are on a path unlooked for and we follow it for a bit loudly saying things like, 'I'm not bothered about this path either way. Are you, Emma?' 'No not me; I'm happy keeping the mountain on my left elbow. Aren't you, Neil?' 'Yes, that's good enough for me; I've no use for a path.' Keeping this up means that

the path continues for some way before it cottons on and then 'Poof!'.

Anyway, paths aside, the walk slowly progresses around the mountain, with the view constantly changing and the terrain altering with each aspect of the hill.

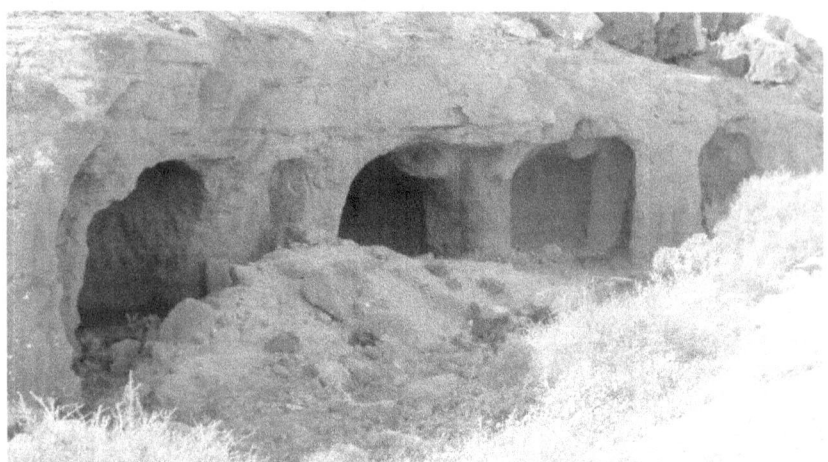

We clamber down a barranco and find we are still ½-way up the mountainside and the going is easy as we pass two smart farms far below us. These clearly make good use of the water from the mountain. Eventually, we can see the car and it is a pleasant stroll back to the warm safety of its steel boxiness.

We repair to Mala and the Arepera for a post-perambulatory cold beer and a *'Why do we do this?'* conversation.

Notes

Incidentally, thank you for buying this book of walks, but...

... for goodness sake, whatever you do: Don't walk the walk. (Just talk the talk like everyone else does.) These walks take you to sights beyond anything you could ever hope to see; where no human eye has ever set foot.

Look at me. I've always loved the Island, but this is addiction. I get out there, away from it all and marvel at a unique and unreal landscape every chance I get. I used to be a jolly, chubby, rotund, sedate gent with umbrella and bowler hat, breathless just looking at a flight of stairs, but now all of that has gone. I've lost stones; my fat has turned to grizzly old leg muscle and I walk up mountains without complaining. I don't want that to happen to you!

Running – that's awful; you can see good, honest distress on the faces of runners. It is just a torture invented to inflict pain on fat people. Runners say it's great when they reach the finish line, but that's like banging your head against the wall – it's nice when you stop.

But walking is deceptive. It's really fun to be striving to pick out a route to the top of the mountain, or to follow a map, or to decipher the ravings of a walking guide author. The work is hard but you don't notice because the barranco is exciting or the mountain path thrilling and then suddenly you reach the corona and look down in awe into the bowl of another volcano, or you struggle to the peak and admire the view of the whole world. (OK, about half of the Island of Lanzarote really, but to me it's the same thing.) It's still great to sit in the Arepera with beer so cold it forms ice in the froth and say how glad we are that it's all over, but we never really experienced the pain in the first place. We take pleasure when we stop banging our head, but we never really noticed the pain when we were doing it. No, don't do it. You'll exercise mightily without noticing the discomfort and have such a fab time that you'll never be able to give it up. So much better to never start than to have to kick the habit later.

El Golfo Montana Quemada Playa Del Paso Circle

This is a 3-hour, hard soled boot walk, not strenuous, with no risk of vertigo, in spite of a 148m peak height. Fine views.

Take a compass, binoculars a map and your stick.

Not remote. This is one of those walks that take us over well-trodden paths where your heart-attack will see you discovered and revived in mere minutes. We prefer *the path less trodden* where when you are eventually found it will be no more than your bleached bones that remain to decorate the scenery, but this is none such.

We drive to El Golfo on LZ704 and park in the large car park on the left. We walk back up the LZ704 until we see a track on the Left with a rubbish bin.

We follow the track marvelling at how it was built. The larva is so rough that it can hardly be walked and tracked vehicles could not cross it. It amazes me how roads are built through that terrain.

We continue, curving right at a farm, pausing only to pat the donkey, and continue until reaching a turning on the left with a remarkable and wholly incongruous gateway. Pause to wonder

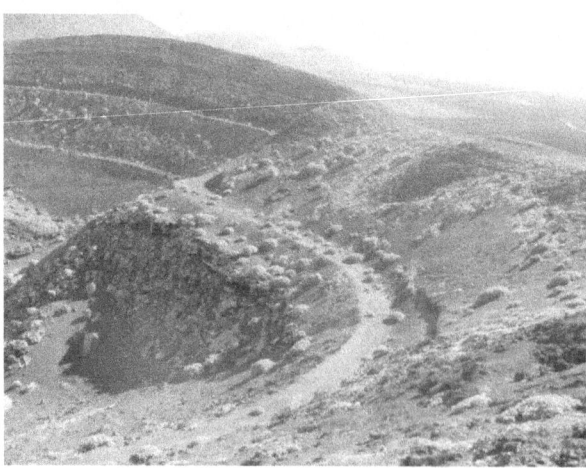

why it is here, and then pass through. A few yards further on we take a faint path right, uphill through the pecon passing stone enclosures, marvelling at how these lava stones lock together in the weakest looking structures but form imperishable structures all over the island.

Suddenly topping the ridge, we fain interest in the view to gain time to recover our breath. In fact the view into the volcano is spectacular and the views backwards show El Golfo and the sea to good effect. *(Nothing to the sea views that are to come, though.)*

We ascend to the peak on our left, to experience the full view and then follow a faint path down to a track half way down the slope. We might pop down to the basin and back up, or not as we decide at the time.

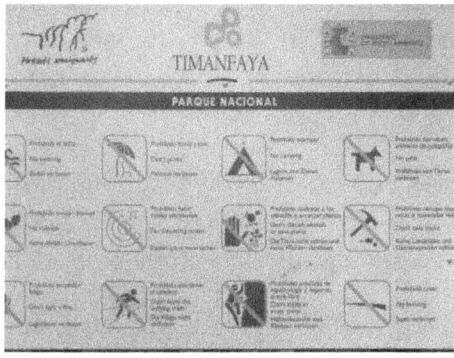

Follow the track to the left, towards a farm house. Keep to the right, so as not to encroach on the house, and we walk past his windmill and down through the pecon to avoid trespassing on his garden. Then back onto the track, passing a national park symbol and a brilliant: *'Do Not..'* sign. This one is so comprehensive as to impress, even on Lanzarote. Essentially, you are not allowed to do anything at all. Nothing! Not even a few things! Whatever you have in mind – don't do it!

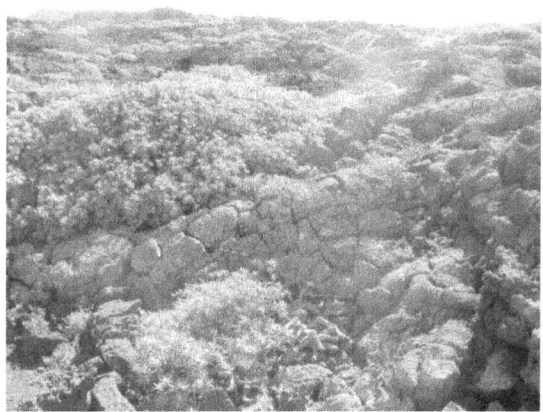

Follow this road; it's a good way but easy walking, until you reach a lovely cove with a black sand beach under a most impressive volcanic cliff. This is a great place for our snack and maybe a quick dip. Didn't bring a costume? Well, it's pretty secluded.

We return back up the track until we reach a sign with a map of this part of the national park. Take a path on our right (South) through the lava to see terrain we will just never find anywhere else. The path is well marked, but rough, so we're pleased we wore hard soled boots. The ground is up and down all of the way and the reason is that we are going over an endless series of lava tubes, measuring from ½-metre up to 10-meters in diameter. In places we can see openings that look like vaulted entrances to a man-made structure. In places we see long tubes, weaving, snaking and dividing on the surface. In places the tube is broken open and we can see it running both ways. In places, larger tubes open up to make remarkable cave systems, although as this is National Park, we're not really supposed to leave the track to explore them.

The path runs close to the edge of the cliff and the sea view is really dramatic. Also we are looking right down onto our beach of earlier. How do you feel about that 'skinny dipping' now?

The path is a fascinating walk, with things you'll not see elsewhere, but it's hard going and continues for an hour or more, so when we return to the village, and find ½-doz fine restaurants offering us our usual post-perambulatory cold beer, we don't hesitate. The sea view is pleasant, so this makes a good time to reminisce and swear that this time we really will be strong and refuse to take any more of these crazy walks.

Continuing on to the end of the village returns us to the car that we left when we so unwisely decided to walk off up the hill.

You know, we only undertook this walk, years ago, because we were all feeling a bit seedy. One of us had a bad knee and giddiness so that he hardly knew what he was doing. The next also had giddiness and hardly knew what she was doing, either. With me, it was liver. I knew it was liver because I had been reading the symptoms on a patent medicine packet and I found that I had them all. It is an extraordinary thing that I have never yet seen a patent medicine advertisement without realizing that I have all of the symptoms described. I think they must target these advertisements terribly well.

I did wonder if it was just clever advertising; but, No. When I looked in a medicine book of the highest repute, I found that indeed it is true; I do have all of those diseases and a good many more besides. It can seem a bit dispiriting to have so many life-threatening problems but if you are careful then the thoroughness of your investigation takes over and your imminent demise from innumerable causes seems to get lost in the exciting study of it all. I found that the Diphtheria was going to be one cause of my eventual failure, but that the yellow fever although classic in its symptomology was in such a mild form that I could survive it for many years if properly controlled.

Anyway, we all thought that exercise and fresh sea air would be just the thing, so we soon found ourselves struggling up the volcano and down to the sea. I'm pretty much cured, but I do find that the others are a bit giddy yet and I'm quite of the view that they rarely know where they are. (With apologies to Gerome)

Notes

The Secret garden

This is a 2-hour, there-and-back, trainers, walk. Easy to find, with strenuous hill sections followed by restful descents, and jolly good for you it is, too! There's no risk of vertigo, in spite of a 100-m height cliff. Fine sea views, and creations, quixotic even by Lanzarote standards.

Bring a memento to leave at the garden. Take a compass, binoculars a map and your stick.

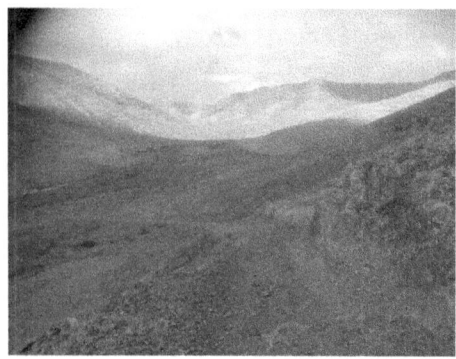

Quite remote, in places. Some walks take us over well-trodden paths where your heart-attack will see you discovered and revived in mere minutes. We love this one because it takes us on *the path less travelled* and when you are eventually found it will be no more than your bleached bones remaining to decorate the scenery.

Take the LZ2, south and turn left at the Lanzarote safari roundabout onto the LZ706 to reach Playa Quemada village on the East coast, two villages South of Puerto Del Carmen. We park on Calle el Toscon, at the South

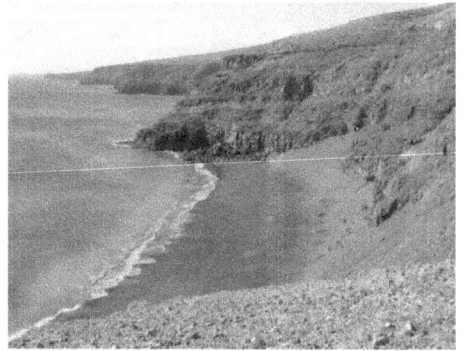

end of the village and walk South.

Leave the village following the coastal path South, zig-

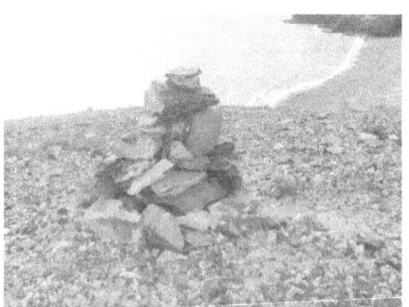

zagging up the hill to the crest. This is a slog, and you should be breathless but just able to talk if you are to benefit from it. Observe the many stone cairns along the way. Some say that these delineate land boundaries and others that they mark the path. Our theory is that each commemorates somebody who died on one of Alan's walks.

From the top, take time to recover under the guise of appreciating the fine view over a deep-blue sea. Further out to sea we can see the large net enclosures and pontoons of the tuna fish farm. We walk down into the valley, where there is a pleasant black sand beach. At low tide we could have walked to this point around the beach, but at high tide - not so much.

We then zig-zag up the next hill. This *effort-followed-by-easy-walking* repeated cycle is doing you the power of good! We cross a barranco and then a second descent takes us to another large beach. Here there are a good range of ruined buildings

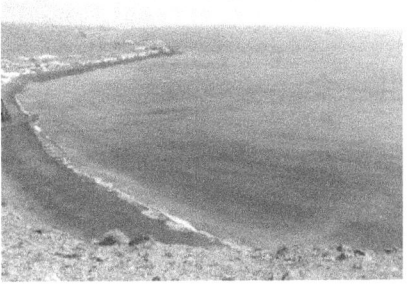

worth a few moments' study, before we struggle up the next hill.

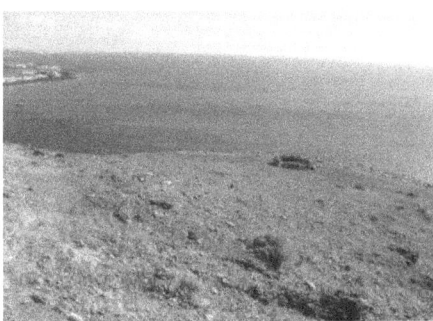

We cross two more barrancos noticing that they exit the cliff at least 50-metres above the sea. In the rain *(and rain it does!)* the water spouts must be a sight to see. We then drop down to the next cove and are just astounded by what we find.

Stop here to eat and drink, and maybe leave a memento to prove that you were foolish enough to undertake this walk and visit the garden. You'll see that many people have done that. This is a nice pebbly beach, secluded in

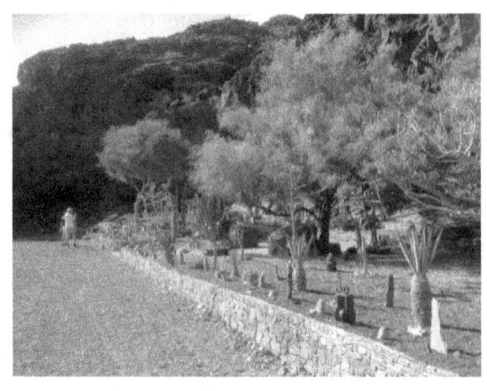

places, so a dip is not out of the question.

Finally, you can retrace your steps. Oddly enough, it is never so

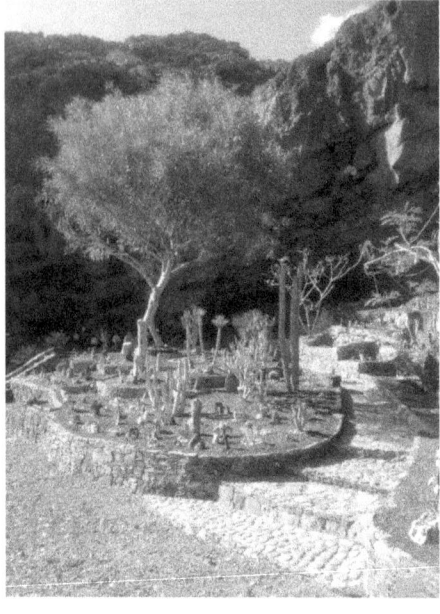

far when you are going back. There are restaurants Playa Quemada offering us our usual post-perambulatory *cold-beer-and-commiserations* and the sea view is very pleasant.

Notes

Perhaps this is a good time to repent; let's swear that this time we really will be strong and refuse to take any more of these crazy Lambert and Wheeler walks. Maybe we should sign the pledge, now...

I the undersigned,

(insert name here)

As attested by those present, do pledge that nevermore will I be persuaded to undertake a Lambert & Wheeler Walk.

I will withstand threats, entreaties and inducements and undertake to hold resolute to this oath until the day I finally weaken.

(Sign here)

Witnesses:

(All those present sign here)

The Pilgrim's Circle

This is a 3-hour, circular, trainers walk, mostly easy to find, with one strenuous hill section followed by long restful descents. There's no risk of vertigo, and remarkable views of the West coast and then the East coast.

Take a compass, binoculars a map and your stick.

It's quite remote, but only in places. Some parts of the walk take us over well-trodden paths where your heart-attack will see you discovered and revived in mere minutes. Other sections are on *the path less travelled* (Frost,1920) such that when you are eventually found it will be no more than your bleached white bones which remain to decorate the scenery.

We walk up the Malpaso Barranco, through 'The little Forrest' and circle around to descend by way of The Pilgrim's Path.

Bring a compass and a map.

Park in Haria, and walk uphill to the West from the Ayuntamiento, turning Left into Call Angel Guerra, and then travell South-West. The road slowly fades away into a track and until eventually it is the gated entrance to a farm and we are obliged to step into the bed of the dry stream. The vegetation on the stream bed is rich and varied as we hop and skip uphill for maybe ½-hour, until we climb stone steps up onto a jeep track.

We cross the track and the Barranco proper is ahead of us. The path is steep but interesting with plenty of vegetation, particularly uphill of the large stone structures built to control water flow. The track is clear and easy to find, but it is necessary to stop to look back and enjoy the view of the rapidly receding Haria (as cover for regaining our breath).

Finally, we reach the top of this climb near a ruined building which has an interesting al jibe with evident channels so that we can see how it keeps full. Although it is no longer in use there is usually 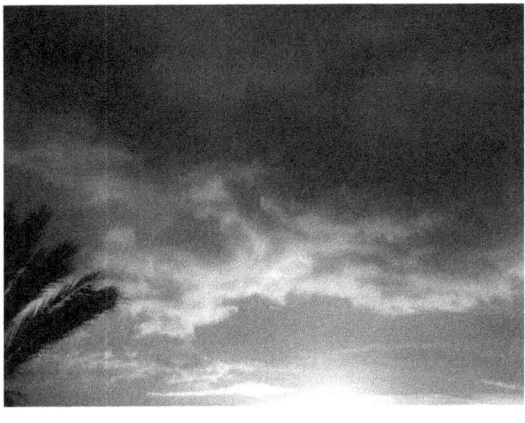 water to be seen in the cistern, showing how well the system works.

Our path continues, crossing over a farm track and we find ourselves under a number of small, olive trees, in an area known as the *Little Forrest*. Here, there are benches and tables, BBQ areas and more importantly a fabulous view over the west coast of the island. We can see Famara beach to our Left and Isla Graciosa to our Right. The walk will amaze us in just a few minutes by showing us an equally fine view of the east coast of the island. Take time to rest, explore and eat sandwiches. This place can also be accessed by car, as we will soon see, and it is the best place on the island to watch the sun set.

Return, later by car, light a barbeque and watch the sun go down.

We leave the Little Forrest walking on a stone track that becomes a cinder track and passes a farm on our left. If we look closely we will see very nice goats, cows and chickens. If we do not look, we will still smell them. Continuing on this path we soon see the Restaurant Los Helechos and our path there is easy enough to follow.

The restaurant is large and serves good food and drink, but the acoustics are dreadful and the best thing is to take our drinks outside and be amazed by the view. Regrettably there are no tables outside, perhaps because it can be just a bit windy. Here we need our map and compass to identify each of the very many settlements before us.

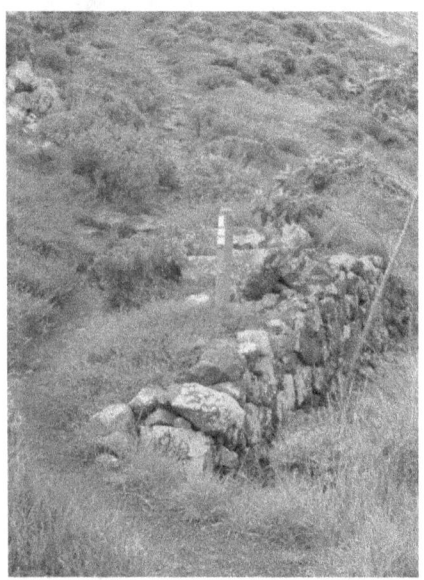

Jarra on board, we walk back onto the LZ10, heading downhill (NW) for about ¼-mile until we see the narrow footpath, clearly signed on our Right, the absolutely delightful 'Pilgrim's Path'. This path crosses the LZ10 over and over and when driving, I had been intrigued by its eight entrances for many years before, under Alan's instruction, I finally walked it.

The path crosses the LZ10 a further three times, passing very closely to the concrete support walls for the road. It is good to marvel for a moment at the civil engineers who built that road. We also see tunnels under the road from time to time to allow streams to run freely as they must when it rains. The path runs down for a good time before joining a track, then a jeep track and then a tar macadam road.

We see a municipal restaurant on our right up a railed ramp in Calejon De La Isleta where it is possible to buy cold bottled beer and very good stew or tortilla. There are also stalls with good fruit, baking, meat and vegetables.

This is a good place to sit and commiserate with one-another about what a dreadfully strenuous morning we've had, but in the long run I prefer to return to The Arepera in Mala to do that. Indeed a super-cold beer and tapas and we'll feel strong enough to swear never to do a Lambert and Wheeler walk again.

Tabayesco circuit

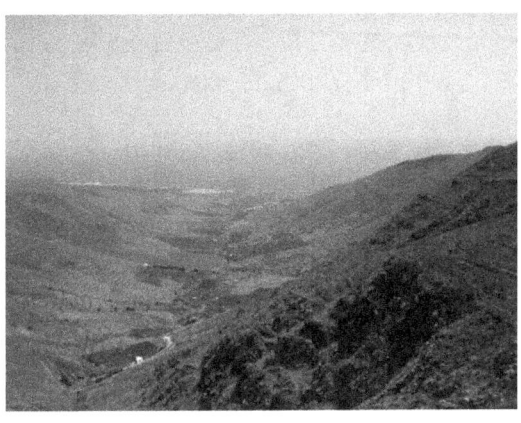

This is a 3-hour, circular, trainers walk, most of it easy to find, with one long hard hill climb through fine country, followed by staggering views and a restful descent. There's no risk of vertigo, and remarkable views of the Tabayesco valley and the East coast.

Take a compass, binoculars a map and your stick.

It's quite remote, but only in places. Some parts of the walk take us over well-trodden paths where your heart-attack will see you discovered and revived in mere minutes. Other sections are on *the path less travelled* such that when you are eventually found it will be, as ever, no more than your bleached white bones which remain to decorate the scenery.

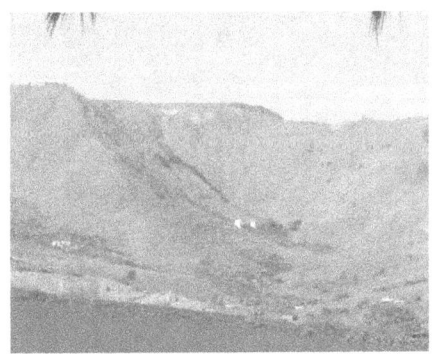

From the LZ206, heading West, fork Right at the bus stop to enter the village. We can park easily in Tabayesco street almost anywhere, but I favour parking beside the bins.

We set out by continuing on this road (West) passing a few houses and the tar macadam soon stops leaving us on a good farm track. From here we can see the Restaurant Los Helechos on the hill and the valley that we will ascend to get there!

The vale is actively farmed and we are likely to see: potatoes, tomatoes, carrots, sweet corn, peas, onions, leeks and figs, before we finish our ascent. Lanzarote is pretty impressive when it comes to low food miles.

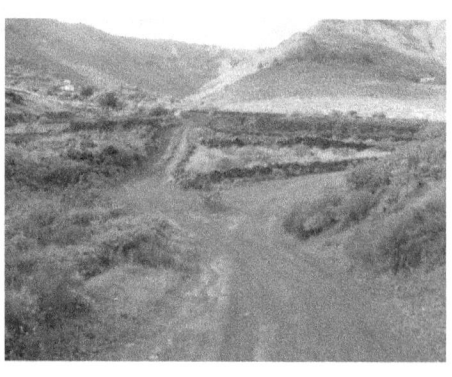

We pass the Finca Natura on out Right and plod steadily on beside an attractive barranco until we reach this 'road island' and turn Right. Right again at the next fork, passing barking (chained) dogs and a fine donkey. The road slowly deteriorates, probably because the steeper it is the fiercer the running water.

Across the valley we see fine terraced farm land and a house with two stories at the roadside and four on our side. Behind us we can see Tabayesco and the sea.

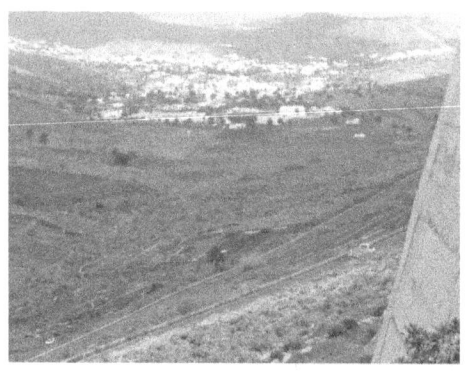

Soon, the road stops altogether. Here, there is a path to the left that clambers up to the LZ206 but our path is to the Right. You could take the left path, and on reaching the LZ206 turn left and in ½-hour you'd be back at the car. However, Alan wants us to go Right, so unless you have a note from your mum its Right.

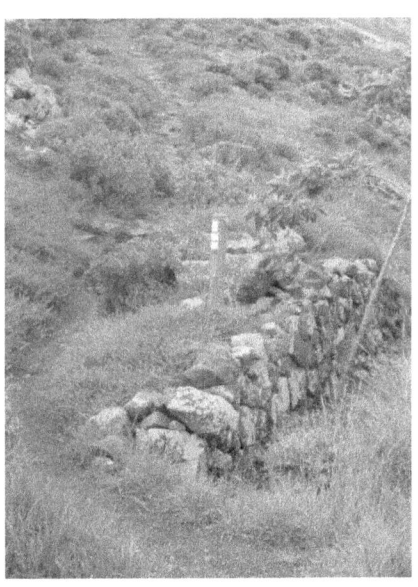

Our path is a clear and delightful walk. It climbs ever more steeply and begins zig-zagging before finally joining the LZ206 where that road meets the LZ10. We turn Right onto the LZ206 and immediately Left onto the LZ10, which we follow for a short period.

On our Left we will soon see the Pilgrim's Path, an even more delightful track *(if a little*

89

steep).

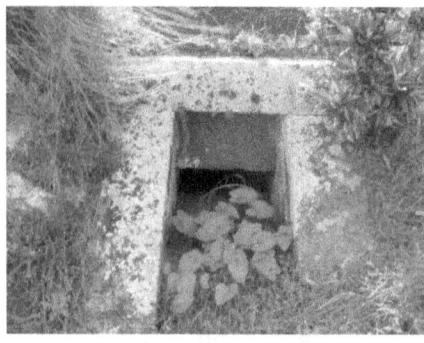

This ancient track climbs steeply over stones worn smooth by endless years of passage.

By way of a rest, we need to repeatedly look behind us and admire the view of Haria.

It is also 'interesting' to spend time admiring the tunnels built under the LZ10 to handle the rain and to marvel at the civil engineers who built that very impressive LZ10 road.

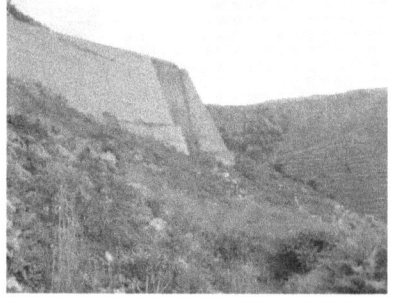

We cross the road once, and continue our ascent. Soon(ish) we reach what appears to be an exit onto the road on a sharp bend, but there is no track on the other side for us to take. This is not an exit, but a gap in the concrete to allow water runoff. Our lot is to continue on this mystical path, (to the Right) and perspire mildly before finding the right place to cross the road for a second time. We zig-zag ever onwards until we reach the road for the third time. This time we do not cross,

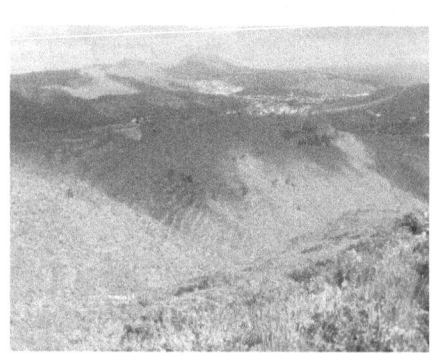

because we can see the Restaurant Los Helechos ahead and the promise of *'Dos jarra pour favour'* lends strength to tired limbs.

Helechos has dreadful acoustics, small chairs and no ambience at all. However the food is good and the beer cold. 'Dos jarra pour favour'. The service is pretty good, too, but the nice man behind the bar repeatedly looks at me and my (undeniably female) companion and assumes that what I really want is to order a 1½-pints.

Now, I say this in the spirit of friendship – Don't tell Emma that she is a girl and therefore can only manage a ½-pint of Cerveza. Not if you want to like to keep your gonads inside your scrotum. This fellow has done it on more than one occasion. Once more and I will not be responsible for the consequences.

Anyway, the view from Los Helechos is unbelievable and there is a mountain plateau ahead and a little to the right that has called to me for years. Today, we're going to go there! We leave the restaurant with the barman intact, (for now) and head South. Ordinarily we don't favour walking on main roads but this one is an exception. We have all driven it and stopped in the various miradors to take photographs, but it has to be walked at least once to know it.

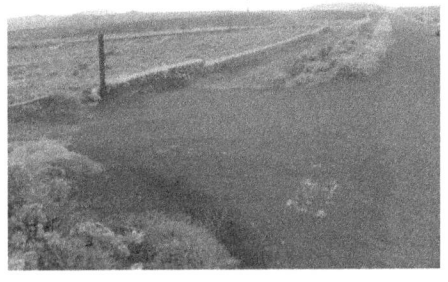

A little after the best viewing point, we see a track on our left.

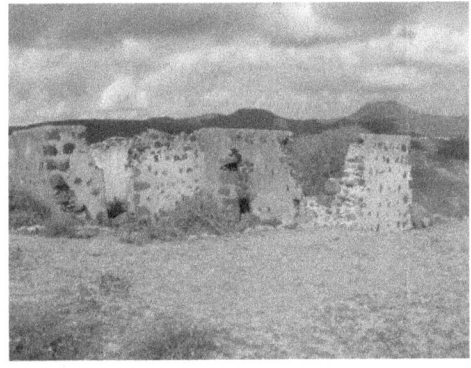

Our track swings to be due West and runs on towards a most wonderfully inviting mountain plateau. Reaching the plateau, we are not a little surprised to find a signpost. We have had to stray for 20-mins from a road to find it. And to make matters worse, the track it indicates is soon to fade away to nothing!

We follow the track as far as it goes and then we are completely abandoned. Luckily you have me; and I have Alan. There really is no track, but the best advice is to head generally downhill clambering fairly easily over the chalky scree. Before long we are offered a ruin as a landmark.

> *There is nowhere like Lanzarote for these ruined farmhouses. In the UK, this one would fetch at least £200K if it had permission to rebuild.*

We make directly for this building and having explored it, find a number of cairns behind it marking out a short section of track, which than (of course) immediately vanishes.

Soon, though, we top a rise and see our goal (Tabayesco) in the valley. Now we have a real landmark and it is a 'simple' matter to negotiate terraces and head downwards, aiming for a loop in the LZ206 road.

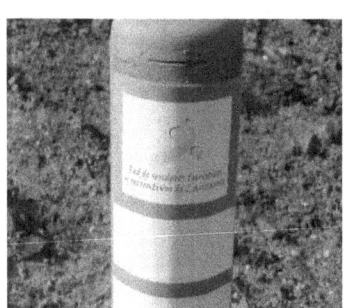

When we see walled fields we pass on their left and strike the road. Possibly the most startling thing to date is that we see that we are standing by a walk marker, indicating that we were on the correct path all of the time. What path? Fair question.

We follow the road around a couple of loops or cut across in a direct line as you prefer.

Soon we see Tabayesco's very own Sociodad so if you need a beer urgently that is your answer; if you can wait, it will be just ten-minutes to Mala and the wonderful Arepera.

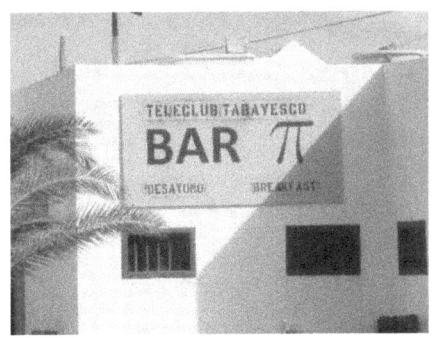

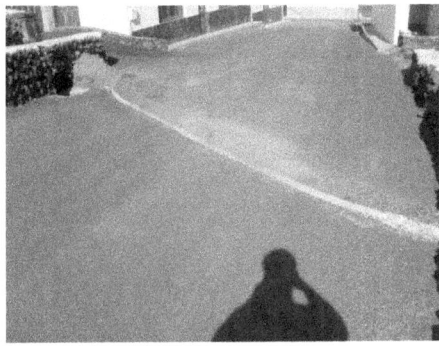

Heading on towards the car, it is interesting to note the rope over the tarmac to direct rainwater from the road into an al jibe on the left-hand-side.

At the Arepera, it is very reasonable to have a very cold beer and tapas, before discussing how to spend time on the island in a way that never means walking anywhere again.

Notes

Tabayesco short-circuit

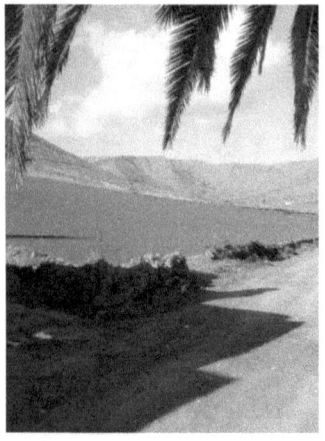

This is a 1½ -hour, circular, trainers walk, easy to find, with one long hard hill climb through fine country, followed by good views and a restful descent. There's no risk of vertigo,

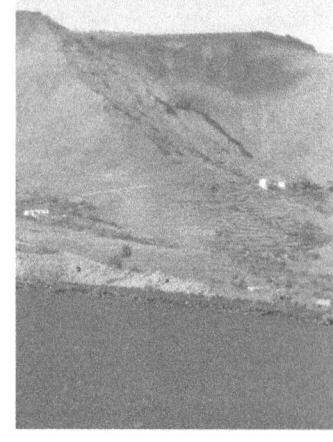

and remarkable views of the Tabayesco valley and the East coast.

It's not remote, but a pleasantly quiet track. May still be bleached white bones territory.

From the LZ206, driving West, fork Right at the bus stop to enter the village. We can park easily in Tabayesco high street

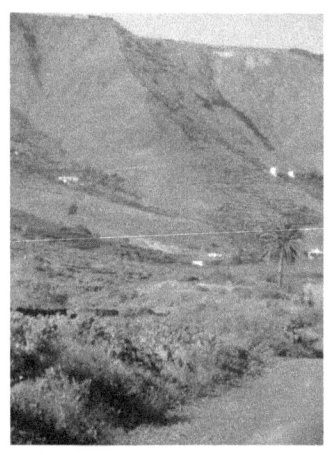

almost anywhere, but I favour parking beside the bins.

We set out by continuing on this road (West) passing a few houses and the tar macadam soon stops leaving us on a good farm track. From here we can see the Restaurant Los Helechos on the hill and the valley that we would ascend to get there if we had taken the full Tabayesco circuit. Well done on your discretion!

The vale is actively farmed and we are likely to see: potatoes, tomatoes, carrots, sweet corn, peas, onions, leeks and figs, before we finish our ascent. Lanzarote is pretty impressive when it comes to low food miles.

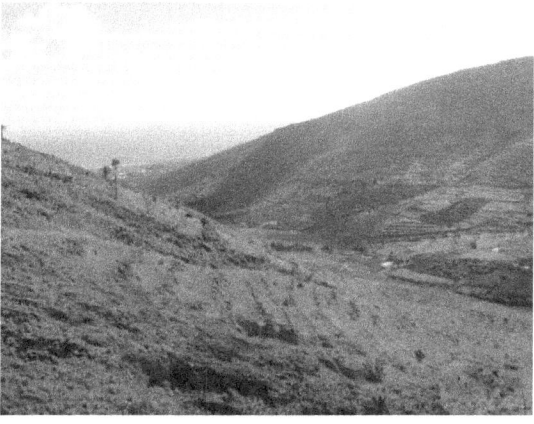

We pass the Finca Natura on our Right and plod steadily on beside an attractive barranco until we reach a 'road island' and turn Right. Right again at the next fork, passing barking (chained) dogs and a fine donkey. The road slowly deteriorates, probably because the steeper it is the fiercer the running water.

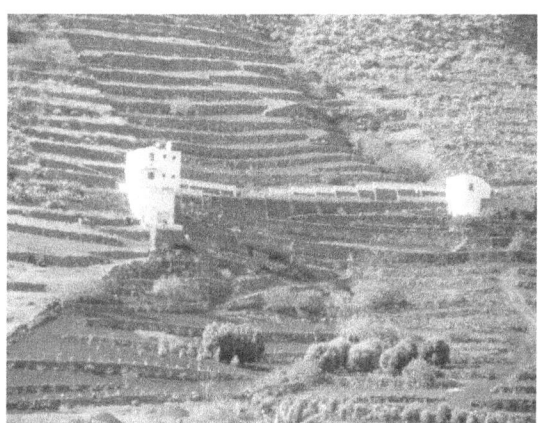

Across the valley we see fine terraced farm land and a house with two stories at the roadside and four on our side. Before long we'll be walking past that house, so can study it more closely. Behind us we can see Tabayesco and the sea.

Soon, the road stops altogether. Here there is a path to the left that clambers up to the LZ206 but our path is to the Right.

You could take the left path and then turn left on reaching the LZ206 and in ½-hour be back at the car. However, I want you to go Right, so unless you have a note from your mother that's what we'll do.

Our path is a clear and most delightful walk. It climbs ever steeper and begins zig-zagging before finally joining the LZ206 where that road meets the LZ10. We turn Left onto the LZ206 and head downhill *(thankfully)* admiring fabulous views to return to Tabayesco and the safety of our car.

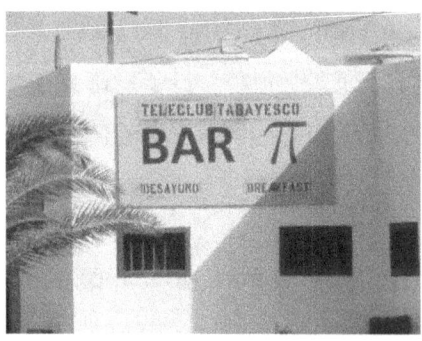

Soon we pass Tabayesco's very own Sociodad so if you need a beer urgently that is your answer. If you can wait, it will be just ten-minutes to the Arepera in Mala.

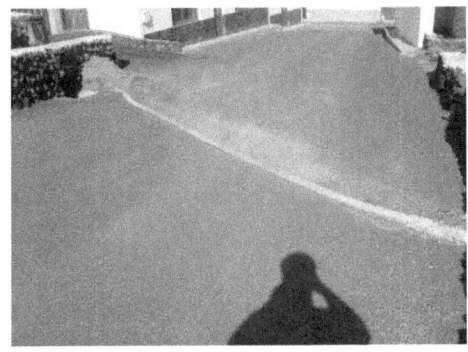

Heading on to the car, it is interesting to note the rope over the road to direct rainwater from the road into an al jibe on the left-hand-side.

At the Arepera, it is very reasonable to have a very

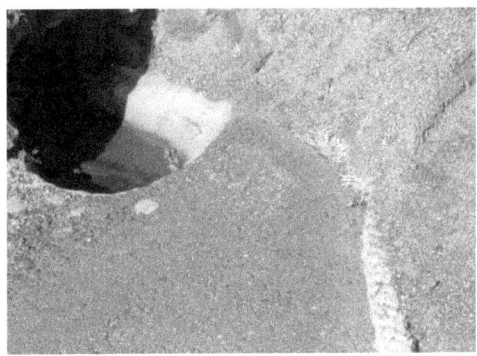

cold beer and tapas, before discussing how to spend time on the island in a way that never means walking anywhere again.

Notes

Femés: better than the Mirador.

This is a ½-hour, up and back, trainers walk, easy to find, with one hard hill sections followed by a fabulous view and restful if picky descent. There is no risk of vertigo, despite remarkable views of the South and West of the island.

If it's not too windy, you have a spare 1/2 –hour and want to see the West coast and the Playa Blanca plain as never before, trot up this little hill and back. Take a compass, binoculars a map to help identify what you see and also your stick.

Taking the LZ702 to Femés, we park outside of the eponymous Femes Café. Where we will take coffee, now, and stew later while benefiting from clean toilets.

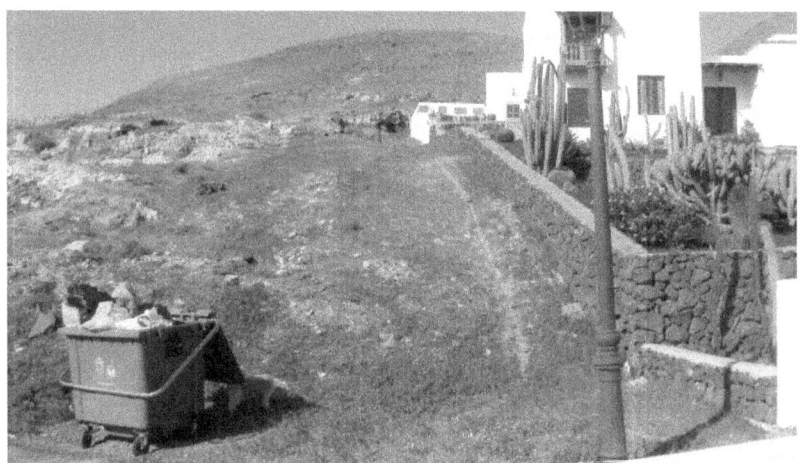

From the Church head uphill, passing the signed Mirador and turn Right onto a brick paved road. Very soon there is a rubbish bin on the Left and a 'path' running up between the bin and a garden wall. Our task is to head to the apex of this little mound. We must not be deterred by the rapid failure of any path; the direction is easy and clear. It may take up to 15-minutes and a good few calories to reach the top. As we top the mound, the entire West coast is suddenly revealed, to the most dramatic effect. The view to the south is also dramatic, looking down onto the Mirador, far below, the entire Playa Blanca plain and then the ocean.

Stay-and-Marvel and then return to the village. We particularly recommend the eponymous Café Femés, for beer and goat stew. It will also be a good place to congratulate yourselves on taking the shortest of the many walks starting from Femes.

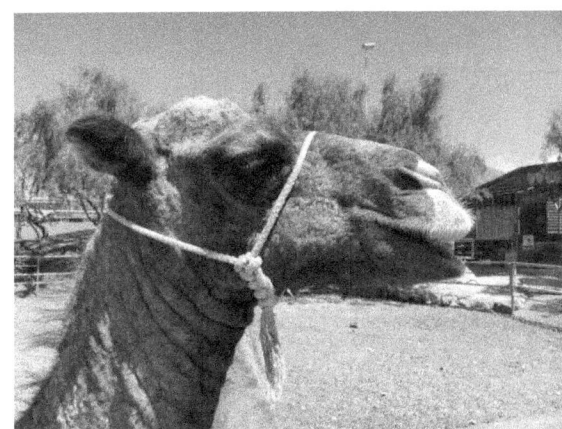

Notes

Femés short, West loop for the intrepid

This is a 1½-hour, circular, trainers walk, mostly easy to find, with one or two hard hill sections followed by restful descents through rough terrain with unreliable paths but clear direction. There's no great risk of vertigo, and remarkable views of the South and West of the island. This is a nice walk around the edge of this very charming town. Take a compass, binoculars a map and your stick.

It's quite remote, in places. Some parts of the walk take us over well-trodden paths where your heart-attack will see you discovered and revived in mere minutes. Other sections are on *the path less travelled* (Frost,1920) such that when you are eventually found it will be no more than your bleached white bones which remain to decorate the scenery.

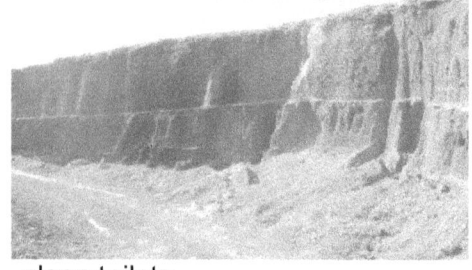

Taking the LZ702 to Femes, we park outside of the eponymous Femes Café. Where we will take coffee, now, and stew later while benefiting from clean toilets.

From the Church head uphill, passing the signed Mirador and turn Right onto a brick paved road. Pass along Calle Juan Caceres Martin, passing Calle Barranco Del Olivo following Camino de Los Pozos. The road curves away and we are following a cinder track around the mountain.

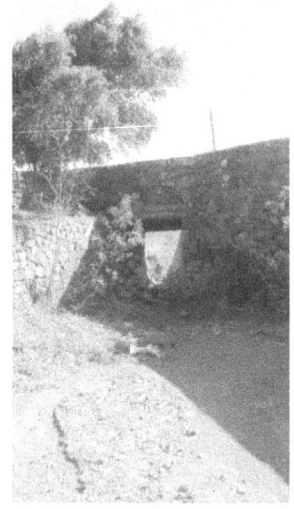

Soon the path offers us a turn on the Left which zig-zags up (and up) the mountain until finally emerging at the peak, near to telephone masts where the entire West coast is suddenly revealed, to dramatic effect. The view to the south is also dramatic, over onto the Playa Blanca plain. Near to the masts is a deserted house and a cave, which has indeed been developed as a dwelling, now abandoned. A very short way back down, we are offered a path on the Left that takes us to a second peak.

From here we would like to head East, to an oasis far below that hosts a roundabout and palm trees. The path there is not always clear but the landmark is always in sight so it presents little difficulty. Much of this part of the descent is in dry rivulets, over occasional dry walls and generally downwards, always facing the roundabout oasis.

If the fates favour us, we will see an artificial barranco ahead of us at right-angles to our travel. We slip into the barranco and follow it down (Right) to its end and there find ourselves at right angles to a path. We turn Left and the path widens out into a level area the purpose of which yet another Lanzarote mystery. Here the track ends. A path on a wall top sustains us for a short while but soon that, too, ends. From here, we can see another wall path down and to our left bordering onto a barranco. A very faint path will get us to it. From the bottom end of this second wall path we cross an abandoned vinyard and pass through a gateway onto the road. We travel on the tar macadam road for a very short way until we see a very deep storm drain which we enter and follow downhill, through a tunnel under the LZ702 and on. until it ends by a 40-foot shipping container.

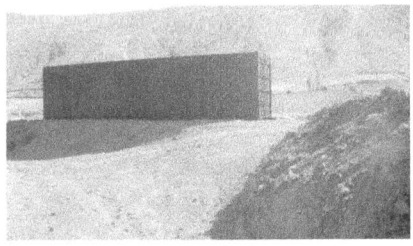

We must stop for a moment's admiration of the lorry driver who delivered the thing to this impossible location.

From the shipping container, we turn Right on a short track that becomes in turn a faint path on the top of a bank that a jeep track and finally a watercourse. The watercourse reaches a low concrete wall which we climb and continue forward along the watercourse which swings to our Right and following it we pass back under the LZ702, climb onto the pavement and trot back to the sanctuary of our car. Thankfully it is just outside the eponymous Café Femés, so toilets, beer and stew are immediately available as part of our celebration that we only took one of the short Femés walks. It could have been so much worse!

Notes

Femés short West loop for Los Anciana

This is a 1-hour, circular, trainers walk, easy to find, without hard hill sections (or consequent restful descents) through easy terrain with reliable paths and clear direction. There's no risk of vertigo, and remarkable views of the settlement; this is a nice walk around the edge of a very charming town.

It is all on well-trodden paths where your heart-attack will see you discovered and revived in mere minutes. This is u our other walks on *the path less travelled* (Frost,1920) wherewhen you were eventually found it would be no more than your bleached white bones which remain to decorate the scenery.

Taking the LZ702 to Femes, we park outside of the eponymous Femes Café. Where we will take coffee, now, and stew later while benefiting from clean toilets.

From the Church head uphill, passing the Mirador and turn Right onto a brick road. Pass along Calle Juan Caceres Martin, passing Calle Barranco Del Olivo following Camino de Los Pozos. The road curves away and we are following a cinder track around the mountain.

Soon the path offers us a turn on the Left which zig-zags up (and up) the mountain. That is hard work, so don't do it! We follow the track gracefully around the mountain passing a few farmhouses and returning to tar macadam roads.

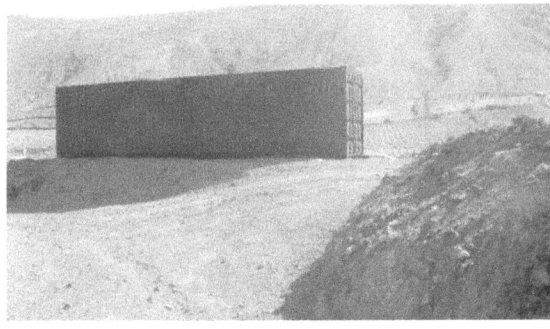

From here you could follow the road back to the car and more importantly the café Femes.

Alternatively we can avoid the road and extend our walk a little, thus:

We travel on the tar macadam road for a very short way until we see a very deep storm drain which we enter and follow downhill, passing through a tunnel under the LZ702, and on until it ends at a 40-foot shipping container.

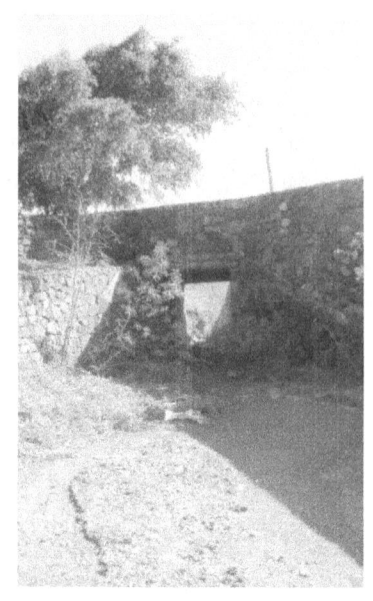

We must stop for a moment to salute the lorry driver who delivered the thing to this impossible location.

From the container, we turn Right on a short track that becomes a faint path on the top of a bank that becomes a track and finally a watercourse. The watercourse reaches a low concrete wall which we climb and continue forward along the watercourse which swings to our Right and following it we pass back under the LZ702 climb onto the pavement and trot back to the sanctuary of our car. Thankfully it is just outside the eponymous café Femes, so toilets beer and stew are immediately available as part of our celebration that we only took one of the short Femes walks. It could have been so much worse!

Notes

Femes long West loop

This is a 2½-hour, circular, trainers walk, mostly easy to find, with one or two hard hill sections followed by restful descents through rough terrain with unreliable paths but clear direction. There's no great risk of vertigo, and remarkable views of the South and West of the island. This is a nice walk around the edge of this very charming town. Take a compass, binoculars a map and your stick.

It's quite remote, in places. Some parts of the walk take us over well-trodden paths where your heart-attack will see you discovered and revived in mere minutes. Other sections are on *the path less travelled* (Frost,1920) such that when you are eventually found it will be no more than your bleached white bones which remain to decorate the scenery.

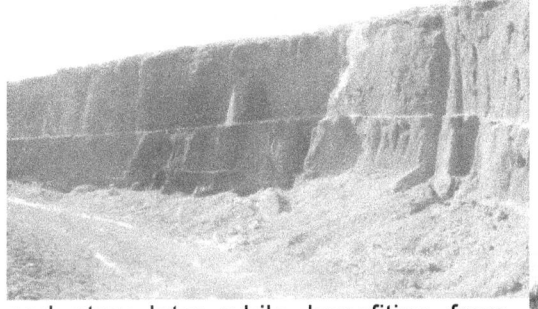

Taking the LZ702 to Femes, we park outside of the eponymous Femes Café. Where we will take coffee, now, and stew later while benefiting from clean toilets.

From the Church head uphill, passing the signed Mirador and turn Right onto a brick paved road. Pass along Calle Juan Caceres Martin, passing Calle Barranco Del Olivo following Camino de Los Pozos. The road curves away and we are following a cinder track around the mountain.

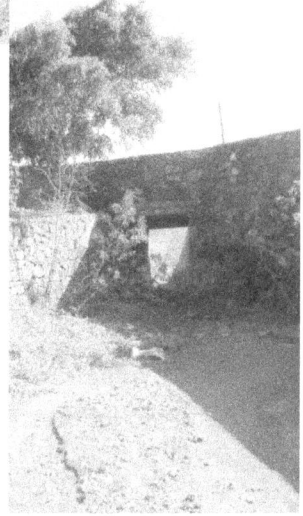

Soon the path offers us a turn on the

right which zig-zags up (and up) the mountain until finally emerging at the peak, near to telephone masts where the entire West coast is suddenly revealed to fine effect. The view to the south is also dramatic, over onto the Playa Blanca plain.

This construction is worth attention. There are houses and caves that reward a few moments and offer respite.

A very short way back down, we are offered a path on the Left that takes us to a second peak. From here a fairly faint North-easterly path takes us down and then up to a second peak and then the same to a third, where a rough road will guide us on the next section.

We look for a sharp turning to the Right which guides us for a 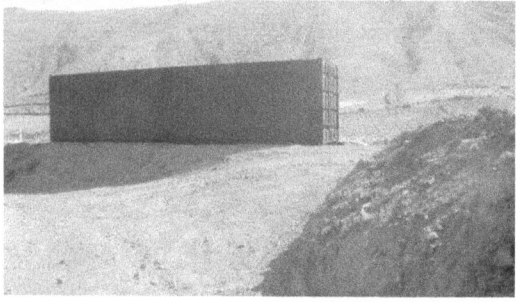 while and then peters out. From here we take a path South-East on the edge of the fields until it reaches a dirt track and thence the road. Trotting up the pavement we reach the bus shelter and then a storm drain crosses under the road. We drop down the steps into the drain, passing under the LZ702, and on until it ends at a 40-foot shipping container.

We salute the lorry driver who delivered the thing to this impossible location.

From the container, we turn Right on a short track that becomes a faint path on the top of a bank that becomes a track and finally a watercourse. The watercourse reaches a low concrete wall which we climb and continue forward along the watercourse which swings to our Right and following it we pass back under the LZ702 climb onto the pavement and trot back to the sanctuary of our car.

Thankfully it is just outside the eponymous Bar Femes, so toilets, beer and stew are immediately available as part of our celebration that it's all over. However we'll never understand why we undertook took one of the longest of the Femes walks. It could not have been much worse!

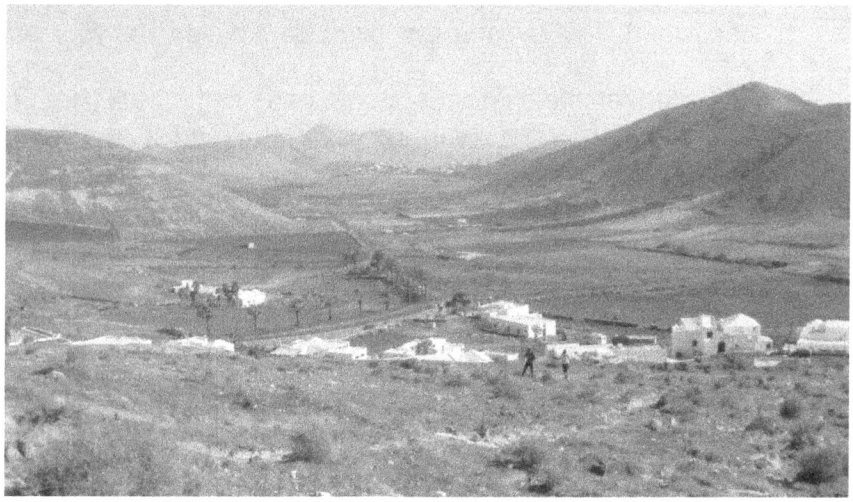

Notes

Goat to Goat, Femés

This is a 3-hour, circular, trainers walk, mostly easy to find, with one or two hard hill sections followed by restful descents through the most fantastic barranco we have yet found. There's no great risk of vertigo, and remarkable views of the South of the island. Take a compass, binoculars a map and your stick.

It's quite remote, in places. Some parts of the walk take us over well-trodden paths where your heart-attack will see you discovered and revived in mere minutes. Other sections are on *the path less travelled* (Frost,1920) such that when you are eventually found it will be no more than your bleached white bones which remain to decorate the scenery.

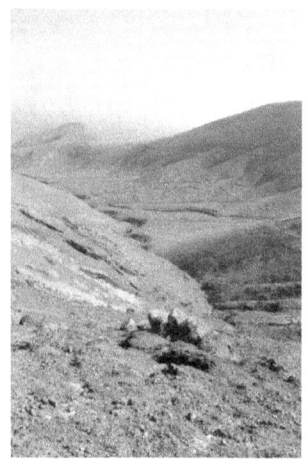

Taking the LZ702 to Femes, we park outside of the eponymous Café Femés. Where we will take coffee, now, and stew later while benefiting from clean toilets.

On the opposite side of the LZ702 from the café we see a zig-zag track up to a building on the horizon.

This is a great goat farm, where we can mingle with these very fine animals if we wish. Dec – March we will see new-born goat kids all around us.

From the peak, there are three paths to be seen. One winds its way around the high mountain to our Right; this is our return path. One follows the crest of the hill on our Left; this is the return from another walk, 'The Femes Barranco and Mountain Crest.'

We are taking the third path, which runs down into the valley. It is easy to see the paths in the distance, but difficult at the start as they are continually eroded by goats.

We scramble down and find the lowest of our three paths, and follow it through a magical valley over the water course until it forks and we select the Right path which will take us up to a mountain saddle, in another ½-hour or so. Lama Del Paso appears on out Left, and if masochism dictates it so, then we can make a short extra loop to experience the view from this peak.

Paso excursion, or none, we continue until we are reassured to find a resting shelter where we might eat, drink and remove pecon from our shoes and shorts. The shelter is not in any way functional *(Affording no actual shelter)* and the decision to put it there is a complete mystery, but it serves very well to reassure us that we are on the correct path.

The path continues to wind around the mountain, affording an ever changing vista until in the pass between Pica Redondo and Hecha Grande we spy another goat farm to our left. We continue to follow the trail to the Right, traversing a path cut into the rock which also carries a black water pipe. The pipe serves to guide us all of the way back to the first goat farm. This is the water supply from one goat farm to the other. It is interesting to consider what a feat this installation was and also to speculate on just how hot the water must be when it arrives. Shower temperature for sure.

Pica Aceltuna (487-metres at the peak) is on our Left as we 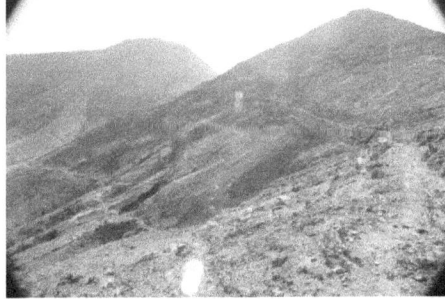 approach the original goat farm and if any spirit remains in us, we can climb to the top and look down onto the Femes Cafe, thinking just how good will be our post-perambulatory beer.

We return to the goat farm, pausing to once more enjoy the beauty of these graceful animals and then trot down the track to the Café. If you want, they will serve you goat stew. By now, we are realizing that there is little hope of a cure; our lot is to walk

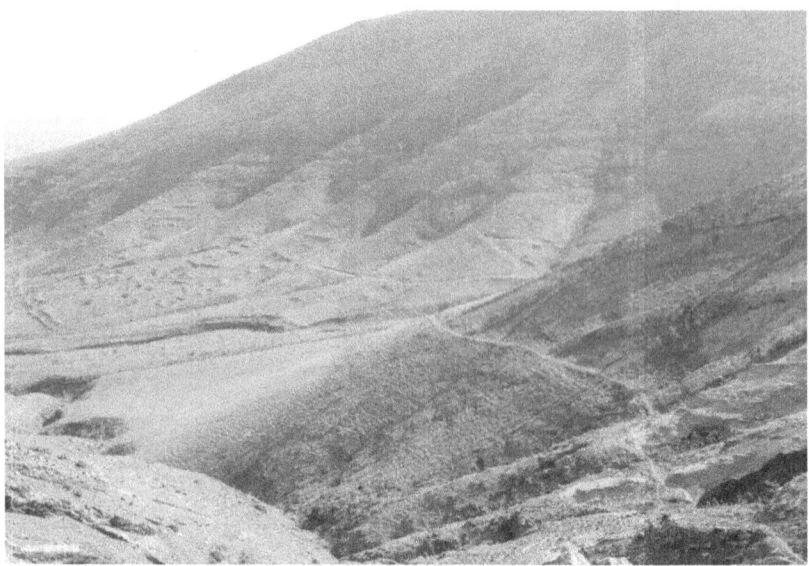

the Lanzarotean landscape for ever more.

Notes

Valley and Ridge Circuit, Femés

This is a 3-hour, circular, trainers walk, only for the intrepid, not entirely easy to find, with one or two seriously hard hill sections after a delightful descent through the most fantastic barranco we have yet found. There's no great risk of vertigo, and remarkable views of the South of the island. Not for a windy day! Take a compass, binoculars a map and your stick.

It's quite remote, in places. Some parts of the walk take us over well-trodden paths where your heart-attack will see you discovered and revived in mere minutes. Other sections are on *the path less travelled* 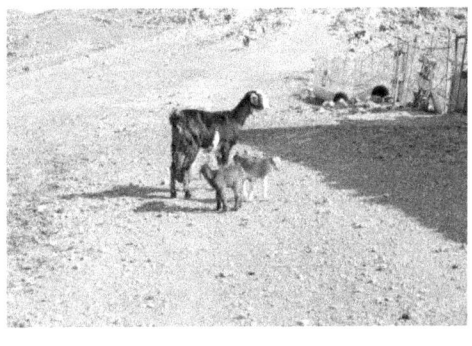 (Frost,1920) such that when you are eventually found it will be no more than your bleached white bones which remain to decorate the scenery.

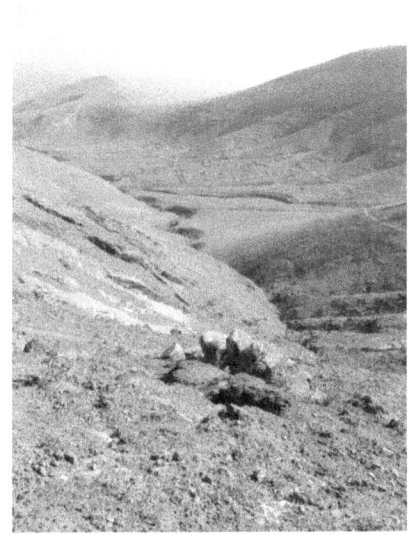

Taking the LZ702 to Femes, we park outside of the eponymous Bar Femés. Where we will take coffee, now, and stew later while benefiting from clean toilets.

On the opposite side of the LZ702 from the café we see a zig-zag track up to a building on the horizon.

This is a great fun goat farm, where we can mingle with these very fine animals if we wish. Dec – March we will even see new-born goat kids all around us.

From the peak, there are three paths to be seen. One winds its way around the high mountain to our Right; one follows the crest of the hill on our Left; this is our return path.

We are taking the third path, which runs down into the valley. It is easy to see the paths in the distance, but difficult at the start as they are continually eroded by goats.

We scramble down and find the lowest of these three paths, and follow it through a magical valley over the water course until it forks and we pass by a turning on the Right path which would take us up to a mountain saddle and Lama Del Paso. We, however continue downwards.

We loop Left to cross a dry stream and then Right to reach a promontory. There is no real path but to the North-West we can see the peak of Pico Oveja and it is entirely possible to pick a path to that. Much panting and the burning of many calories brings us to the peak. Here we are rewarded by yet more fabulous viewing. A little to the West involving a degree of decent, we can reach the ridge. The path is not always clear, but it is reasonably easy to follow the crest of the ridge and eventually achieve the safety and comfort of the goat farm, and thence *beer-and-sympathy* at the eponymous Bar Femés.

Notes

Montana Cuervo

This is a 1-hour, trainers, walk, not remotely strenuous, with no risk of vertigo. Fabulous to experience the inside of a volcano.

This is coach-potato country – not at all remote. A well-trodden path where your heart-attack will see you discovered and revived in mere minutes. It is beloved of coach parties, so selecting the best time of day is important but the gap in the corona that admits you onto the floor of the volcano is one of the best.

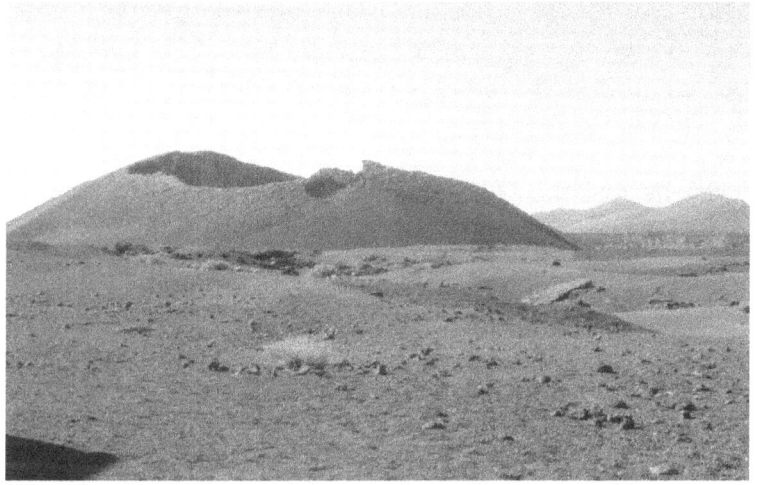

We take the LZ30, which runs from Teguise to Mozaga and on towards Uga and near to Masdache we take the LZ56, North, for a very short way until we see a large car park on our left.

A very good path has been created to take us to the volcano and it is clear and easy to find. When we reach the mountain we can turn left or right, circumnavigating the mountain in either clockwise or anticlockwise direction. Each is as good as the other, but note that the entrance to the volcano is a short way to our right. Whether we want to get there now or later rather depends on which is least likely to see us coinciding with a coach party. The good thing is that the coach trip sees people rush in, photograph each other and rush out again as quickly as possible to reach the next shop on their itinerary. So, with a little patience we can always get this mystical enclosure to ourselves and such is the ambience inside the mountain that we really do want to be alone there.

The walk around the volcano is really very engaging and needs regular stops just to marvel. The path takes us into lava fields that are as good as we would find anyway and very easily accessed - unlike some to which we might take you.

Having communed with ourselves inside the volcano, gazing up at high mountain walls, and walked through fine volcanic lava fields, we reach our return track. From here, there is a clear path up to the corona which is quite inviting, but vertigo cannot be ruled out and the signs clearly do not encourage this climb so we will not either.

If it was just me, I'd go straight on to climb Montana Negra, now, leaving the car where it is and doing enough puffing and panting to feel that I'd had a respectable day of exercise. From that fine mountain peak there is a fabulous view down onto Montana Cuervo.

If that's too much for you, there is a fine Sociodad in Mancha Blanca. However, that being the case, I will not want to hear grumbles. This was not a walk enough to raise a sweat.

Notes

Montana Negra

This is a 1½ -hour, trainers, walk, pretty strenuous, but with only minimal risk of vertigo in spite of a 515-m peak height. Fabulous views over the volcanoes of the South and a remarkable view down onto the famous Montana Cuervo.

Take a compass, binoculars a map and your stick.

Quite remote. Some walks take us over well-trodden paths where your heart-attack will see you discovered and revived in mere minutes. We love this one, though, because it takes us on *the path less Travelled* and when you are eventually found it will be no more than your bleached bones that remain to decorate the scenery.

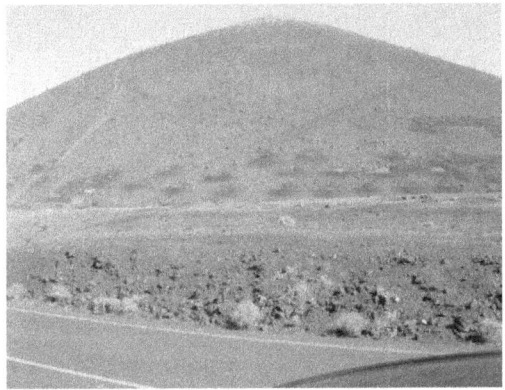 We take the LZ30, which runs from Teguise to Mozaga and on towards Uga and near to Masdache we take the LZ56, North, for a very short way until we see a large car park on our left.

Our mountain is on the right and we can see the path options running to the mountain peak.

Walking to the mountain path is simple and we start our ascent next to a building that is still in use for agricultural purposes. We struggle upwards along a path that keeps forking and dividing. This is a good, literal, example of *'Many roads up the mountain'* and it doesn't really matter which we choose. Each goes to the same place. Some circle the mountain gently and some ascend rather more directly and each is fine as long as we select one that is generally uphill. After a while we reach the bowl of the volcano, and the general greenery in the bowl is quite remarkable.

Like so many mountains here, it suddenly becomes quite lush and verdant. This greenery continues right to the peak. In autumn, the sedums are in flower, as are the geraniums and later the marguerites making this a colourful spot. There is also a decent grove of olive trees. From here two 'arms' reach up to the peak. Either arm makes a satisfactory route uphill. From the peak, we can look down on the Montana Cuervo and beyond it to a vast array of mountains in all directions. A while with a map and compass will see us identifying mountains and habitations all around.

Descent, when we are ready again can be conducted in many directions, noticing Caldera Colorada just to our North.

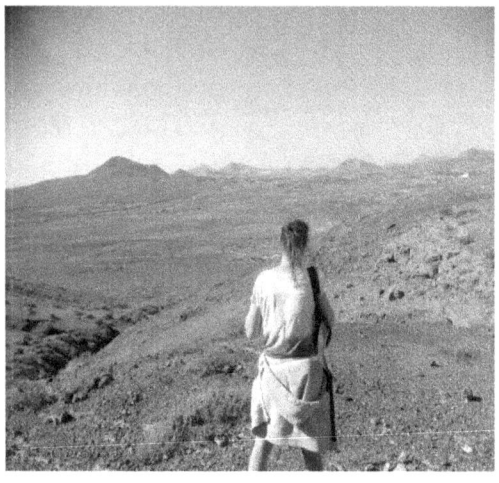

Were it me, I would now trot over and try Caldera Colorada, but if you prefer then it's a Post-perambulatory cold beer at the Sociodad in Mancha Blanca, where you might swear never to attempt Colorada, but we both know you'll weaken, and give it a go.

Notes

This is a 1-hour, trainers, walk, not remotely strenuous, with no risk of vertigo. Fine way to see a 'Bomb' and read up on the making of a volcano.

This is coach-potato country – not at all remote. Well-trodden path where your heart-attack will see you discovered and revived in mere minutes. Beloved of coach parties, so selecting the best time of day is 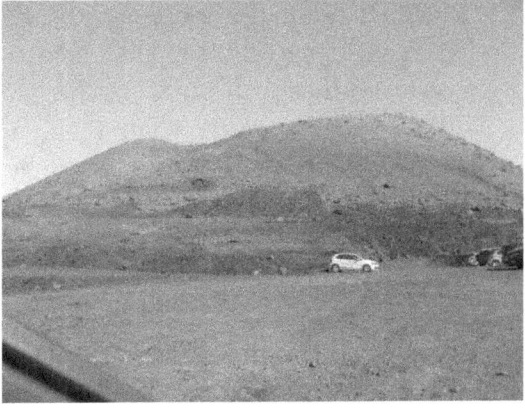 important but the walk is pleasant and the explanations of the volcano is one of the best.

We take the LZ30, which runs from Teguise to Mozaga and on towards Uga, and near to Masdache we take the LZ56, North, a short way until we see a large car park on our left. Our mountain is a little further on the right again with a car park.

We can walk either clockwise or anticlockwise and there is no benefit to either, save that we can avoid a crowd by choosing whichever option they eschew.

Throughout the National Park walks we find photographs, maps (usually incorrectly orientated) and descriptions of landscape that would embarrass even a geography teacher. This landscape it the most dramatic, exciting, thrilling, stirring, stimulating, inspiring, electrifying and motivating scenery we could ever hope to find. *(And I only end there because my stock of synonyms is so limited.)* However, *the powers* have a way of writing copy to make the most exciting vision ever seem duller than the worst geography lesson you ever slept through. Perhaps it's better in the original Spanish. Anyway, the boards

117

on this walk are the exception so allow time to look at them. They explain the creation of a bomb, meaning a rock that congealed in the sky and fell to ground, leaving you grateful if you were standing somewhere else. Near the sign is an excellent example of the phenomenon.

Further around, the creation of a volcanic corona is explained. You will have noticed that most of the volcanoes face in the same direction. *(If you haven't, then look around you now.)* Nearly all have a high 'head' and a pair of 'arms', curling around towards a large gap, looking faintly like a cartoon character. All point in one direction and that is because much of the corona is formed from pitched ash and this is affected by prevailing winds and… Anyway, if you read the explanations, this will all be made clear to you.

While walking, you will see a path slanting up through the pecon to the corona. This is a worthwhile effort affording a fine view of the inside of the volcano and also of the Montana Negra, behind you. However, this is a tough climb, the ground under foot not as firm as you'd like and vertigo a serious issue. So, if you pass that by, that's probably wise.

Having walked full circle, you will have had a pleasant stroll. If you're now ready for a climb, scramble up Montana Negra, next door.

If not Negra, then it's a *Post-perambulatory-cold-beer-for-wimps* at the Sociodad in Mancha Blanca. Here you might swear never to attempt Negra, but we both know you'll weaken, eventually, and give it a go.

Notes

Montana Los Rodeos

This is a 2-hour, trainers, Near-circular walk, not very

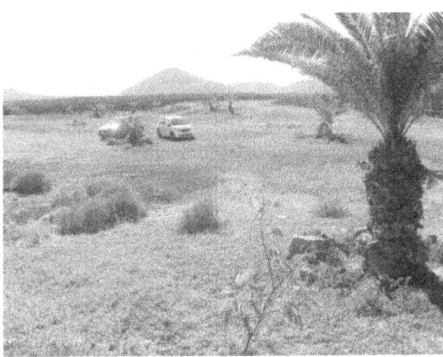

strenuous, with no risk of vertigo, even on the optional 454-m peak height. Fabulous views over the volcanoes of the South and a remarkable stretch of lava. Take a compass, binoculars a map and your stick.

Quite remote. Some walks take us over well-trodden paths where your heart-attack will see you discovered and revived in mere minutes. We love this one, though, because it takes us on *the path less Travelled* and when you are eventually found it will

be no more than your bleached bones that remain to decorate the scenery.

Park in the delightful oasis towards the North end of the LZ56, Just to the South of Mancha Blanca.

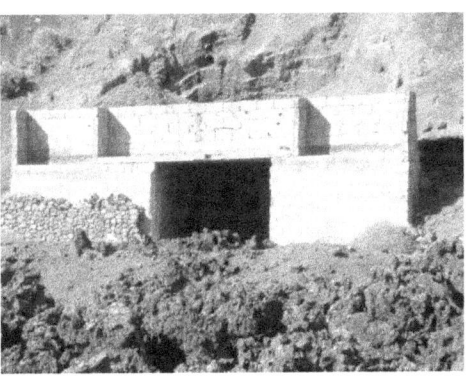

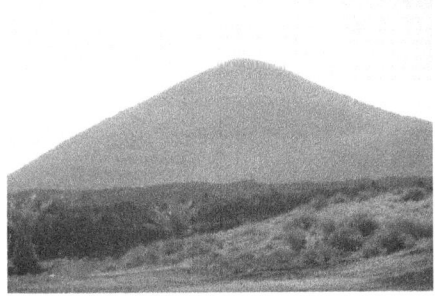

Walk along the left of the paths, which is the one not stone surfaced and soon you will be puzzled by a hobbit hole in the hill on your right. This is a block structure and although this is an extensive construction it only actually encloses a space big enough to park a car. Perhaps the rest of the structure is to give protection against rocks and water tumbling from the mountain.

Continuing along this path takes us through some impressive and very varied lava fields. In places looking as though it has just run, cooled and set yesterday.

The path is a good one, progressing steadily to the mountain. At the base of the mountain we are able to turn left or right. Each is as good as the other so if there should be other walkers, we always take the route that ensures the greatest solitude.

Anyway, turn left or right *as you like* and process around this double-peaked mountain. Offered further forks, we just take the route that holds us closest to the mountain.

This is another twin-peaked mountain and when we are at the furthest point in our circuit we can climb to the lower and thence to the higher peak. Not too tough in the main and it gives us a magical view.

From the high peak there is an option *(I'm afraid)*. We could retrace our steps to the far end of the circuit and continue our mountain circumnavigatory route. This is probably a good option as the lava is varied and well worth seeing. Alternatively, though, this peak is the volcano's 'head' and the usual two 'arms' curve out to the North and it is perfectly possible to walk down either of these arms to the ground and we find ourselves at the original and philosophically troublesome T-junction, with just one section of track left to travel before returning to the blessed sanctuary which is our car.

From the car, the nearest cold beer is in Mancha Blanca at the Sociodad. Sat in the bar we wonder why we did not just park in the lovely oasis, take a few snaps, and have a little nap in the car. *Maybe next time; nobody will know.*

Notes

Uga short Loop

This is a 1½ -hour, almost-circular, trainers walk, easy to find, with one long hard hill climb through fine grape country, followed by good views and a restful descent. There's no risk of vertigo, in spite of a 507-Metre peak, and remarkable views of the vineyards and the myriad mountains of the South.

It's not remote, but a pleasantly quiet track. May still be bleached white bones territory, in places.

From the LZ206, driving West, take the LZ30, North and park at the footpath, signed on your right in a few hundred metres.

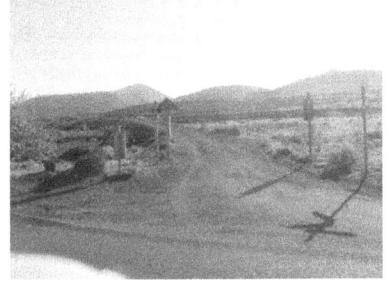

We park near the entrance to the track. This is a section of the Orzola to Playa Blanca route, so adequately signed. It is also intensively farmed, so the road is pretty good.

Head eastwards and upwards, through vine basins and fig trees.

The road is raised a good height in place for no reason that I can identify.

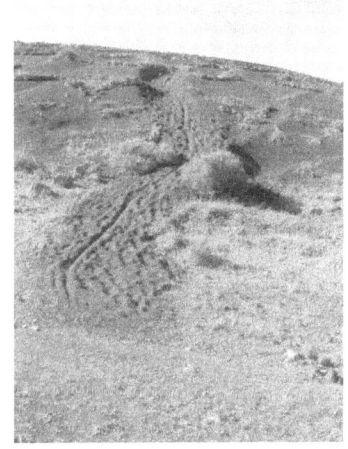

And up, and up, *(and up)* pausing regularly to draw breath and feign interest the endless vineyards across the valley we remember how much good this is doing us. In the autumn, the figs are abundant and although small are absolutely delicious.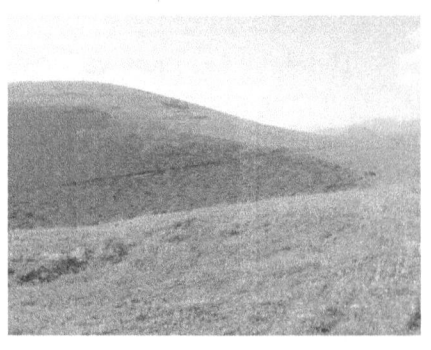
Most are left to rot as you will see by looking at the ground under the three, so I feel OK about scrumping a few. However, they can have an unwelcome effect for one so far from a toilet, so for myself I am modest in my sampling. As we get, thankfully, near to the top three car tracks appear on the right and after those a foot path on the right

Following the path steeply upwards we strike a jeep track, which we can follow around to our Right, to reach a first, a second (higher) and a third (highest) peak, each offering a different fine view.

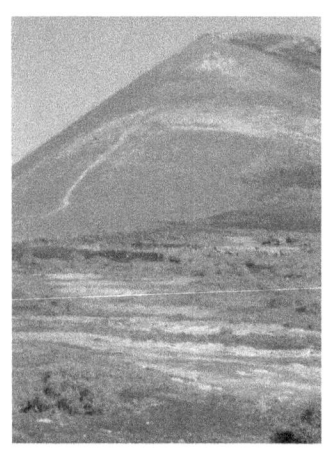

Recovered and refreshed, our track loops on around to the left passing a complex of al jibes and a ruin before finally regaining our original road/track at the mountain pass. From here, the view is East as well as West so different again.

Across the track, you might be tempted by the near-perfect cone of Montana de Guardilama. This is a steep path, with a mild risk of vertigo and will take about an extra 40-mins, but the view is fab and otherwise our walk from here is a gently downhill trek to the refuge of the car, so maybe it is OK to go.

From here, having popped up to the peak and back *(or not –
nobody will judge you)* we take the track back to the West,
towards Uga and the safe haven which is our car. This is a very
gentle coasting down all of the way and takes remarkably little
time. Do pause, though, to look in detail at the ever-changing
view across the valley and Uga nestled between the hills.
Notice a very odd circular hole surrounded by a smart wall in
the centre of Uga. You will probably want to know what it is and
my answer is *'So do I'*. Later, if we follow signs to the Mercado
we will find this excavation and a careful study will leave us
none-the-wiser.

Attaining the protection afforded us by our car, Uga is clearly
the nearest source of post-perambulatory (purely medicinal)
alcohol. Even for me, Mala and the Arepera are too far to go.
So in Uga, we eat, drink remove pecon from\intimate places
and congratulate ourselves on selecting the shortest of the
three Uga walks.

Notes

Uga Loop

This is a 2½ -hour, circular, trainers walk, easy to find, with one long hard hill climb through fine wine country, followed by good views and a restful descent. There's no risk of vertigo, in spite

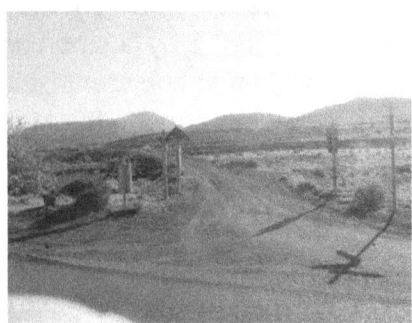

of a 507-Metre peak and there are remarkable views of the vineyards and the myriad mountains of the South.

From the LZ206, driving West, take the LZ30, North and park at the footpath, signed on your right in a few hundred metres.

We park near the entrance to the track. This is a section of the Orzola to Playa Blanca route, so adequately signed. It is also intensively farmed, so the road is pretty good.

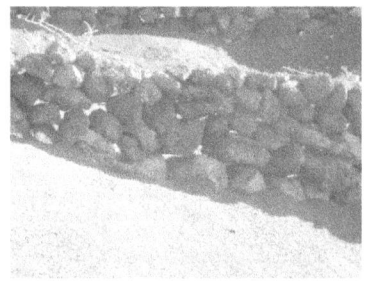

Head eastwards and upwards, through vine basins and fig trees.

It is interesting to study the stone walls giving wind protection to the vines. These are totally frail,

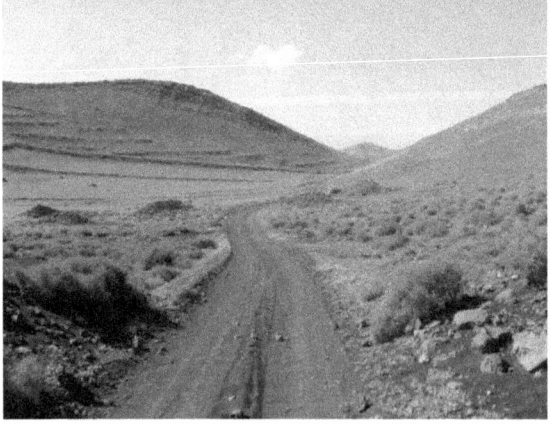

single stones, one on another and look entirely fragile. The nature of the volcanic rock is such that it just locks together and lasts for ever. The pods on the beach are the same, of course.

124

The road is raised a good height in place for no reason that I can identify.

And up, and up, pausing regularly to gaze at the endless vineyards across the valley and remember how much good this is doing us. In Autumn, the figs are abundant and although small are absolutely delicious. Most are left to rot as you will see by looking at the ground under the three, so I feel OK about sampling a few. However, they can have an unfortunate effect for one so far from a toilet, so for myself I am cautious.

After much effort and no little perspiration, we reach the mountain pass and are rewarded by fabulous Easterly views. Here, however, we have a cunning plan for adding still more climbing to our route!

We will take the jeep track on our Right between two low stone pillars. Circling South and looping around to our Right, passing the ubiquitous ruined farm and a complex set of al jibes we reach the mountain's peak (Montana Tinasaria). Here, we pause to eat, drink, curse the pecon in our shoes, and enjoy the view.

Head on, downwards along the track for just a short way we reach another slight plateau. From here we can see an (only mildly precipitous) track down the side of the mountain to join a jeep track that heads West. Following the jeep track, we pass between fine mountains and emerge to gain a good view of Uga and our destination.

Occasionally in the winter, this route can display a continuous mass of flowers, resembling a wild-flower meadow.

Continuing, we see a strange concrete structure on the hill to our left, which turns out to be the run-off for another failed reservoir. The position should allow for collection of a great deal of water; the positioning is perfect and the catchment area extensive. However the rock is porous and we can see from the vegetation that it has never held water; not even for a short period. Reaching the road, we turn Right and walk, uphill, to the safety of the car.

Uga is the nearest source of post-perambulatory (purely medicinal) alcohol. Even for me, Mala and the Arepera would be too far to go. Eat, drink and congratulate yourselves on selecting the second shortest of the three Uga walks.

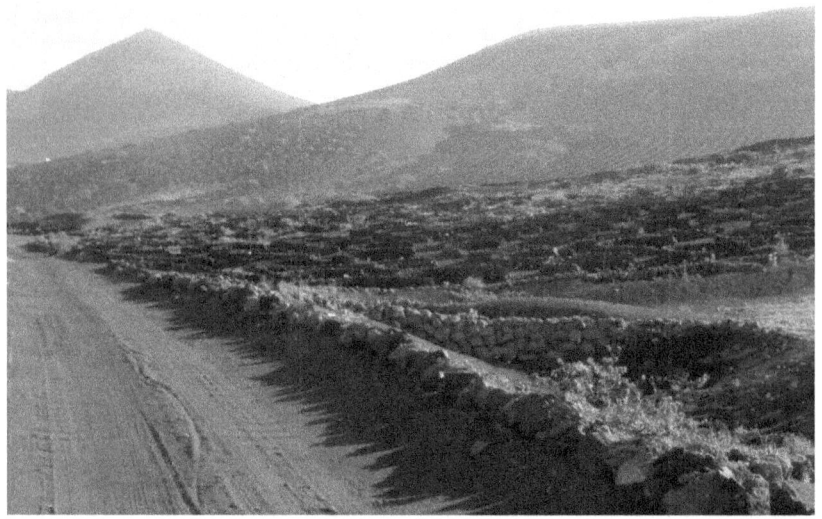

Notes

Uga long Loop

This is a 3½ -hour, circular, trainers walk, easy to find, with one long hard hill climb through fine country, followed by good views and a restful descent. *(OK, and a few more slight climbs)*. There's no risk of vertigo, in spite of a 507-Metre peak and remarkable views of the vineyards and the myriad mountains of the South.

It's not remote, but a pleasantly quiet track. May still be bleached white bones territory, in places, though.

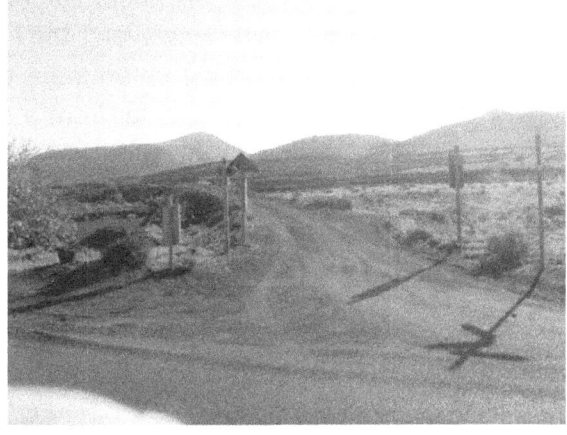

From the LZ206, driving West, take the LZ30, North and park at the footpath, signed on your right in a few hundred metres.

We park near the entrance to the track. This is a section of the Orzola to Playa Blanca route, so adequately signed. It is also intensively farmed, so the road is pretty good.

Head eastwards and upwards, through vine basins and fig trees. We study the stone walls giving wind protection to the vines. These appear totally frail, single stones, one on another

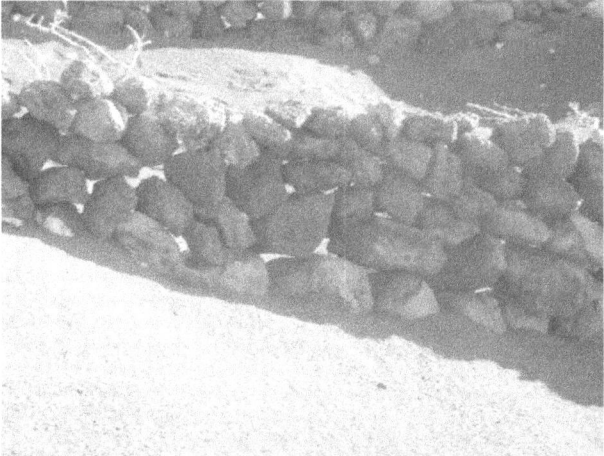

127

and look entirely fragile. The nature of the volcanic rock is such, though, that it just locks together and lasts for ever. The pods on the beach are the same, of course. The road is raised a good height in places, also for no reason that I can identify.

And up, and up, pausing regularly to gaze at the endless vineyards across the valley and remember how much good this is doing us. In Autumn, the figs are abundant and although small are absolutely delicious. Most are left to rot as you will

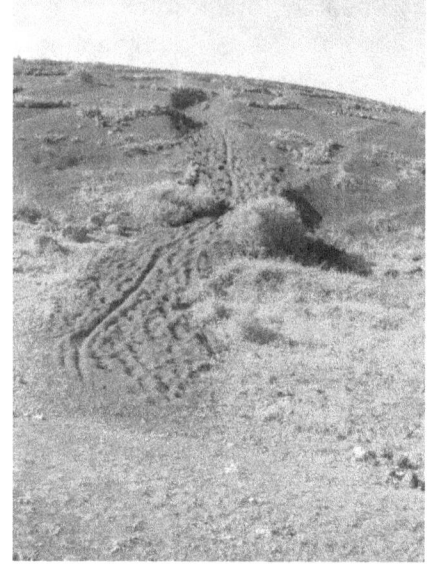

see by looking at the ground under the three, so I feel OK about sampling a few. However, they can have an unfortunate effect for one so far from a toilet, so for myself I am modest in my scrumping.

As we get, thankfully, near to the top three car tracks appear on the right and after those a path on the right.

Following the path steeply upwards we strike a jeep track, which we can follow around, to reach a first, a second and a third peak, each offering a different fine view.

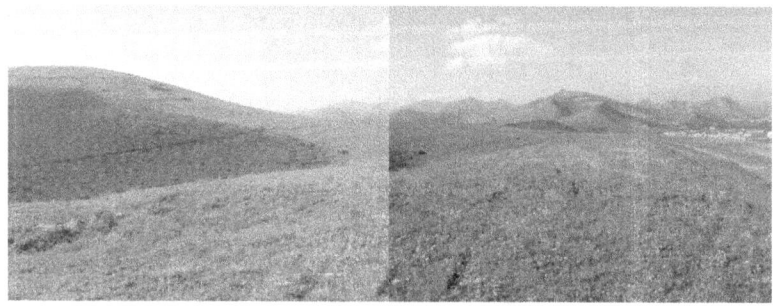

Recovered and refreshed, our track loops on around to the left passing a complex of al jibes and a ruin before finally regaining our original road/track on the mountain pass. From here, the view is East, so different again.

Now, we head on East, downhill passing a farm entrance and then turning right to head towards the sea. On our left we are passing some of the best gardens to be seen on the island. On our right we are impressed to see a small football area with real grass.

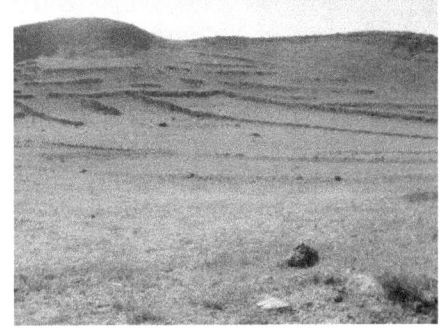

Onwards and downwards, we reach a cross-road and turn Right. We pass a mass of al jibes. Each has a large concrete water collecting area, rather than a channel to catch the mountain run-off. Were there

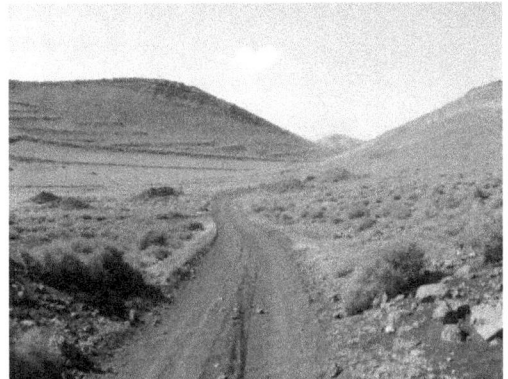

contest for the most al jibes per acre, this would surely take it.

Just before reaching a roundabout, near the signpost, we strike off to the right on a jeep track that follows a line of pylons. It feels good to be away from the tar macadam again. We pass an isolated farm with a busy windmill, and continue on *(and on)* until we reach a cross-road. Here we turn Right, pushing uphill to reach a mountain pass where we swing Left. Following this track, we pass through and between several mountains to emerge into what can be a charming flower meadow in a wet autumn/spring. There is a pleasant little volcano on our right worthy of a slight detour although the basin is not deep.

Continuing, we see a strange concrete structure on the hill to our Left which turns out to be the run-off for another failed reservoir. The position should allow for collection of a great deal of water; the positioning is perfect and the catchment impressive. However the rock is porous and we can see from the vegetation that it has never held water at all, even for a short period. Nothing.

Reaching the road, we turn Right and walk, uphill, to grasp the emotional crutch which is our car.

Uga is the nearest source of post-perambulatory (purely medicinal) alcohol. Even for me, Mala and the Arepera is too far to go. Eat, drink and commiserate with yourselves on selecting the longest of the three Uga walks. Still, at least it is over, now.

Notes

This is a 3-hour, trainers, walk, pretty strenuous for the final hour, with only minimal risk of vertigo in spite of a 400-m high cliff. Fabulous views of the cliffs, the beach the salt pans and Isla Graciosa.

Take a compass, binoculars and your stick.

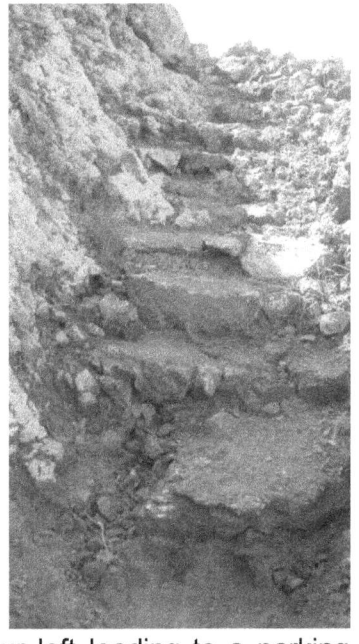

This is a walk down a well-trodden path so your inevitable heart-attack will see you discovered and revived in mere minutes. Not, *'the path less Travelled'* (Frost,1920) where when you were eventually found it would be no more than your bleached bones that remain to decorate the scenery.

From the South edge of Ye, we take the back road towards Mirador Del Rio quickly passing Finca La Corona on our right and finding a stone paved turning on our left leading to a parking place. Here the lava is rampant, forming fascinating outcrops and valleys worthy of photographic deliberation. Cacti grow prolifically here; many showing signs of goat predation.

The stone paving guides us to a mirador (viewing point) where the faint hearted sit and marvel, but we intrepid types just step over the edge and follow fantasy steps cut into the cliff face. The path zig-zags wildly descending steeply but fairly safely down and down *(and down…)*.

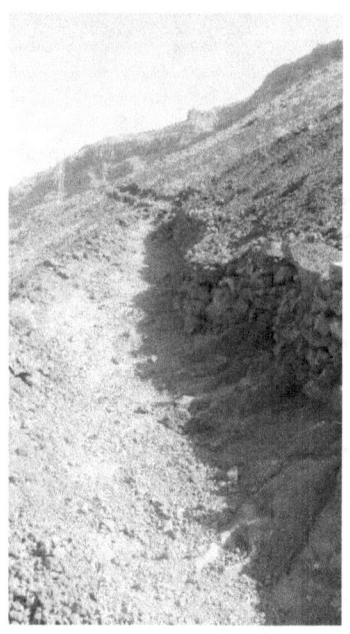

After considerably more than ½-hour's descent the path gently levels out, we go over a cross-road and another ¼-hour will take us to the sea shore. Usually, this is pretty deserted so that a quick dip is fine whether we remembered swimsuits or not. From here if we want to extend we might want to walk North over to the Salinas Del Rio and see how salt is collected as well as gazing up at the Mirador Del Rio wondering whether people paying their euro to use the high-power telescopes found our skinny dipping to their liking.

With or without the salinas excursion, we return to the cross-road. From here, should we wish, we could take the path South (*another optional excursion?!*) and walk under the cliffs for some way before returning to the cross-road to tackle the final ascent. So far the walking has been easy, but this last haul involves a little effort and we will be glad of our sticks. Perhaps an hour of steps will see us back at the cliff top where we can give superior looks to the faint-hearted-types still sat on the wall at the viewing point.

A few minutes back along the track see us at the car and we can drop the *cool* act and collapse into the welcoming embrace of our car seats.

From here, the Ye Sociodad is the nearest post-perambulatory cold beer but we will want to maintain our air of superiority so cannot indulge our usual competition about which of us hates walking the most.

> *'Well of course walking for me is particularly difficult because one of my legs is shorter than the other'.*

'One leg shorter than the other? That's nothing! One of mine is longer than the other and everyone knows that's much worse.'

Ha! A couple of mismatched legs is nothing; I've been walking for years with two arthritic hip joints'.

Only two arthritic joints? Luxury! I've had Arthritis, Rheumatism and Gout in every joint of my body for ninety-years and a broken ankle for the last ½-mile'.

'Arthritis, Rheumatism and Gout in every joint for ninety-years and a broken ankle. You lot don't know what trouble is. I was born with no joints in my legs at all and had to ....'

Anyway, this time there can be no post-mortem and no grumbles. We just sit loudly saying that it was all 'A *bit of an anti-climax really'* and, *'Almost too easy'* and, *'If it wasn't about to get dark we'd trot down and up again just to make the outing worthwhile'.* You can never be sure that there isn't one of those faint-hearted types sat at the next table in the bar.

Notes

Caldera Caldereta and Blanca

This is a 2½-hour, hard soled, walk, not especially strenuous, with some (optional) risk of vertigo on a 460-m high corona. Fabulous views across the national park.

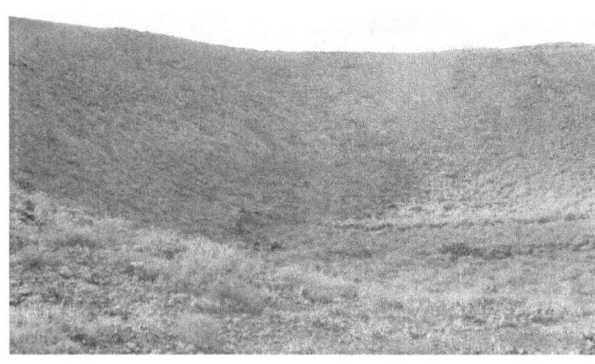

Take a compass, binoculars and your stick.

This is a walk down a well-trodden, official path so your heart-attack will see you discovered and revived in mere minutes. A not entirely easy walk you do have to work at it in places. Not this time, 'the path less Travelled' (Frost,1920) where when you were eventually found it would be no more than your bleached bones that remain to decorate the scenery.

We park in Mancha Blanca, on a westerly track off the LZ67, where there are several official parking spaces, just North-East of the Visitor's Centre.

We take the obvious westerly path, reading dull explanations of lava along the way. The lava is spectacular and ever-changing and worth the walk all on its own. How it is that 'The *Authorities'* manage to make the information boards so desperately dull is a mystery. They are informative in the manner adopted by the very worst geography lessons you ever experienced. The path is good, wide and clear but stony so hard soles and a stick are a must. Frequently we see an interesting lava feature and must allow time to marvel at it all as well as just paying photographic homage.

The path is a bit too good and we fear the coach potato, but fear not; it becomes difficult, unclear and slightly dangerous before long, so our sense of adventure will be more than sated.

The path first reaches; a smaller mountain at just 326-metres, but fabulous. It is possible to scramble up the scree to the corona but not essential because there is more to come. Rounding the volcano, we see that there is a 'ground-level' entrance to the volcanic bowl with al jibes and ruins at the entrance. It is essential to round the bolder and walk into this bowl. Stand in the centre and rotate, for full effect. This may be one of our favourite volcano basins. Exiting the Caldereta entrance, we notice a sort of bridge in front of us and inspection shows that it is covering another al jibe and one so efficient as to be usually full, even after many years of neglect.

Our path requires us to walk gently upwards along the side of the Caldereta and once we are about half way up the side we see that the path strike off to our right through lava. *(Again, we use the term path rather loosely.)* The trick is to remember that we are heading for Blanca and pick our way forward. Sometimes there is no path at all and then we suddenly stumble upon a clearly pathified section. This *path – no path* section takes us over lava quite unlike that which we saw earlier and soon drops us onto a real path where we turn right(ish) before, by a huge boulder, we see a path diagonally up the side of the Caldera Blanca itself.

Climbing to the corona is achieved by way of a clearly visible path, which occasionally makes use of a water channel such that we are walking in a 1-metre deep trench. Broaching the corona we are treated to the most impressive view into the bowl ahead of us and behind us another view over many miles. Those who experience vertigo can enjoy this very wide ledge and its unthreatening views and take a picnic at this point. The map&compass come into play here, identifying towns and mountains all around us before we send the vertigo sufferers back down the path to the sanctuary of a collection of inexplicable corrals from where it is possible to turn Right and rejoin the outbound path. Retrace to the car.

Less sensitive souls can navigate the corona either way around; both are possible. We then drop down a steep 'path' at the Westernmost point to the base of the mountain and take a path North and then East to gain the sanctuary of the collection of inexplicable corrals mentioned above. From there it is

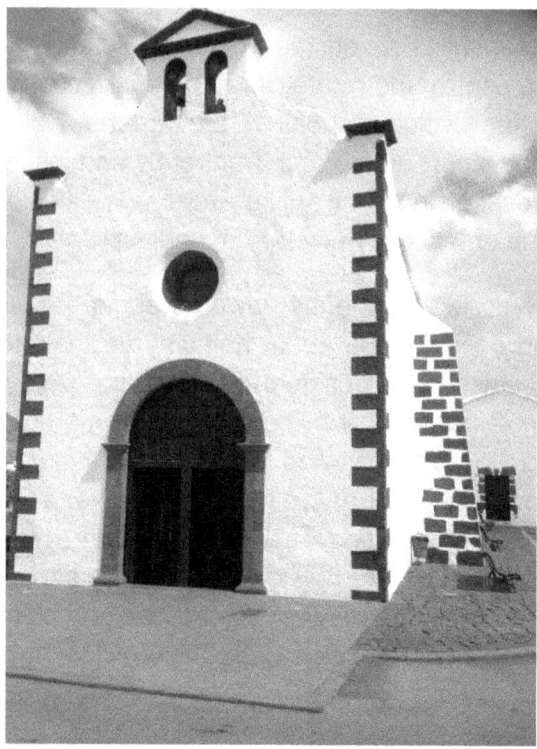

possible to continue East and rejoin the outbound path at the al jibe we saw when exiting Caldereta.

Retracing our steps we achieve the sanctuary that we have missed since so foolishly leaving the car. The nearest restorative bar is in Mancha Blanca, which also boasts a supermarket if our water has been exhausted.

Notes

Montana Ubigue, Nazaret - for the timid

This is a 1½-hour, trainer, walk, not especially strenuous, with no risk of vertigo on a 308-m high corona. Nice views across Nazaret and Tahiche and the mountains to the West.

Take Map&Compass and your binoculars.

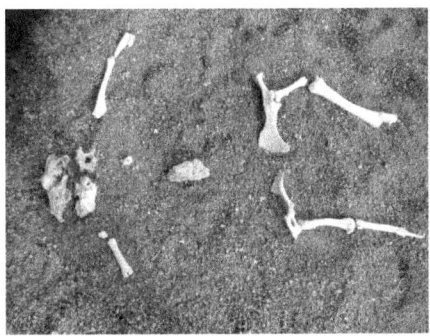

This is a walk up and down a jeep path so your heart-attack will see you discovered and revived in mere minutes. Not this time, *'the path less Travelled'* (Frost,1920) where when you were eventually found it would be no more than your bleached white bones that remain to decorate the scenery.

An entirely easy walk over clear tracks and on an old corona that is greatly softened by time. There are no rocky outcrops; no precipitous slopes. Good for the timid who still want to look down from the corona. You do have to work in the initial climb, but after that it's a coast.

We take the LZ10, South fromTeguise and just before it reaches a left-hand bend with protective rails, we take a road on the right. We follow that road into Nazaret over a cross road and as it deteriorates we find an informal parking area on the right, bordered with boulders.

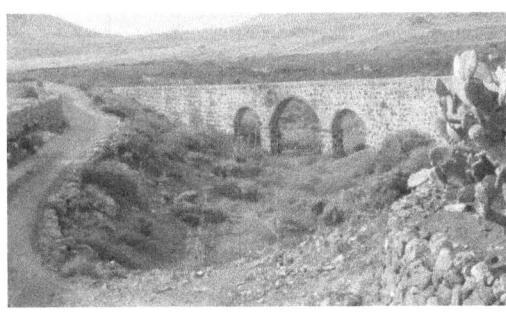

We continue walking along this road, forking Left, signed casa Nazaret. We pass a farmhouse and the track dips to pass through a gulley with an ornate bridge to our

Right. The purpose of this bridge is a mystery, if you know the answer, *(Gunga Din)*, then you are a better man than I. The path continues; we ignore a fork to our Left (our return route) pass the barranco and see a jeep track running up the side of the mountain.

> *(Personally, I'd not take my Morris Minor up that track but as we keep seeing Lanzarotean drivers take vehicles to the most unlikely places.)*

The climb is a bit of a puff, but that is why it does us so much good. We reach the first peak and the view to the Left of mountains Zanzamas and Maneje are very pleasing. We 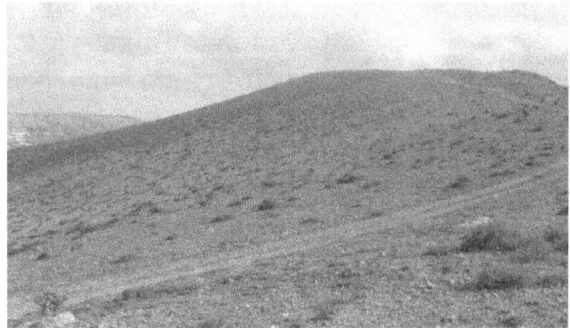 progress to the higher peak, marked with a cross. From here the view of Tahiche and beyond to Costa Teguise are good or in the other direction, over Nazaret. To the left we see the volcano's basin and the barranco.

Refreshed, watered, fed and relieved of intrusive pecon, we can make our way down the second arm of this volcano, still following the jeep track. This rejoins our earlier route and we recognise the turning that we passed earlier. The track gently returns to the car. Having had such an easy outing so far you might want to run this last bit *(not!)*.

Returning, there are ample bars for post-perambulatory beer and tapas, but we prefer to experience delayed gratification by waiting until we reach Mala and The Arepera. In whichever bar we sit, it behoves us to applaud each-other for the wisdom displayed in selecting such a nice short walk.

I guide like this you when you are faced with a choice each option having equal benefit lest you find yourself unable to decide. In a deterministic universe, we imagine that we have free-will, but in fact all actions are determined by that which has gone before. So, we will make a left/right (yes/no, up/down, etc) decision based on our set of experiences to date. Since we have only one past (one make-up and one set of experiences) we can make only one decision at any time and any sense we have of 'free-will' is illusory. What we will do in any situation is 'predetermined' by what has happened before. An interesting consequence of this is that if we have no relevant experience, then we may be unable to decide at all.

Determinism dictates that a donkey equidistant between two identical feed mangers will be unable to favour one over the other, unable to decide, and will starve to death. (Of course, this is a thought experiment; no real donkey involved. Like Schrödinger's cat; no cat was rendered simultaneously alive and dead just to demonstrate quantum theory) (For a full explanation of quantum theory and how it clashes with general relativity, see appendix 1).

You, faced with two equal choices and no information to guide you may prove ill-equipped to make a decision. (For more on determinism, see appendix 2.)

Notes

Thank you

Thank you for coming with us. We've had you in mind at every step and we really do feel your company on each walk. Write to us: nwheeler@brookes.ac.uk

And remember, if you feel that you would like to take more walks with Lambert and Wheeler, there are people at your Local Health Centre with therapies to cure you. Otherwise, when you feel the urge for a Lambert and Wheeler Walk, just lie down in a darkened room and it will pass off.

Appendix 1

Hah!

If you think you are going to get a full explanation of quantum theory and how it clashes with general relativity in a walking guide you're going to be sorely disappointed.

Appendix 2

Extracted from 'A Letter from Elvis, the writings of a remarkable pig.

Meredith Farm Campsite,
Llancloudy
Herefordshire
HR2 8QR

A letter from Elvis - 4

Hello everybody. Elvis, it is, again.

Once more, I must thank you so much all of those who have written to me and special thanks for all of those apples and pears. As always, I will reply to all of your letters, but in the meantime:

John: Yes certainly, tea bags are delicious;

Michael: it may be muddy, but there is nothing like it on a hot day;

Ms C: I think it would work if you marinated it for a day first, but you need to be careful about the ingredients;

Frances: Really you should not think of doing it like that.

Again, I am free for a few moments. I do appreciate The Royal Arms for minding Dear Old Neil for me. He'll be back after his usual $\frac{1}{2}$ pint of foaming ale.

Now, as I go about my day and in this heat, I get to thinking. And what I think is this. We all imagine we decide what to do for ourselves. Some humans call that 'free-will', but I don't think that it is true. (OK thinking and humans seldom go together but pigs think a lot and I am trying to bring you along a bit.)

You see, it feels as though I can decide whether to come or go and what to eat first and so on, but I'm not sure I really do decide. I think it may be an illusion. Every decision I make is not simply up to me to make a random move. I inevitably base each choice on what I know, what I have experienced in the past, what I'm like and so on. So, as I have only one set of experiences and one make-up, there can actually be only one choice that I can make in any situation. That is to say that I could not decide other than I do because of the life I have lived so far. I have lived the life I have lived and my actions can only be as they must be as a consequence. My present is 100% determined by my past and my future is determined by my present. I can only do as I must.

I imagine I choose what to do; it feels like I do, but because that choice is entirely based on the things that went before then it is not up to me but a result of my history.

This is a funny sort of feeling. It feels like I make all of my decisions, but logically, I think that I cannot be doing that. So I checked into it. A human called Hume and before him, Laplas had much the same thought, though neither of them could say it as well as a pig would have. Then another human called Skinner said even so we do somehow retain free will.

I don't know. I will think some more and let you know.

I must tell you about the goat on the cooker incident, too, but not now because I hear Old Neil's car. I'll sign off because Old Neil does not know about my letters. No point in telling him – there is very little in them he'd understand.

Good night all of you.

Elvis.

Appendix 3

Extracted from 'A Letter from Elvis, the writings of a remarkable pig.

Meredith Farm Campsite,
Llancloudy, Herefordshire
HR2 8QR

A letter from Elvis - 6

Hello again everybody. Elvis, it is... again.

Once more, you have written to me and a special thank you for all of those apples.

As always, I'll reply to all of your letters, but in the meantime:

Michael: If you were to add some grit, I think you'll find it drains more and the problem will go away

Janet: All humans have a degree of fragility. I don't think you should worry about it.

Frank: If you blanch them first and then let them cool, you'll find the flavour is much better.

Frances: Really! I won't tell you again!

As before, I am free for a few moments, with Royal Arms minding Neil for me. He'll be back after his usual, "Half-pint of your best foaming ale, please landlord".

The summer has gone, and autumn is here, turning cold. I want to take this opportunity to tell you something well known to every pig, but humans insist on not believing it.

There are two kinds of things, Animate things and Inanimate things. I am using animate here to refer to things that are intelligent, sentient, mobile and control their destiny: Pigs, Dolphins, White mice and, to some extent, Humans.

Inanimate things cannot move themselves or really 'do' anything. They are not sentient, not aware, not mobile or in any way in control of their (non) lives.

And all of this makes them mad! And they hate the animate things, because they see it as so very unfair. As a result, they wage a non-stop war against the animate world, focussing their ire mostly, I am sorry to say, on Humans.

I will explain all of this to you, 'though it might take more than one letter. You will see that it is all nonsense and of course it is, but you will also see that it is all true and it obviously is. We won't win this war, it is all stacked against us, but at least you'll know the truth.

To start showing you the position, I'll just give examples and you will begin to see the truth. It is given to inanimate objects to become invisible for short periods of time. That is why when you look in a drawer for something that you know for a fact is there you will not be able to see it. It can become invisible at that moment. It cannot actually become invisible at will; it has to gain the energy for that trick from you. In particular, it gains the energy from your distress. You will say a rude human word. You will say that 'I KNOW IT IS IN THERE'. You will look again and again you will have no luck. You will not see it. You admit defeat and go out and buy another. Then when you look in the drawer again, later, there it is, right on the top, clear as day, saying 'Did you want me?' All innocent, like. Of course it doesn't speak really; it is inanimate. But it says it anyway. You no longer need it, so there is no energy available to support the invisibility so you can now see it perfectly easily.

You think that you have won in the end, because you bought the replacement spanner and did the job. But No! It won! It did not seek to prevent you for ever from fixing your tap because it couldn't hope to do that; it is enough that it inconvenienced you. And, By George! Did it inconvenience you!

You load yourself up with things to carry them to somewhere and the door swings shut on you. Why? Just to be awkward! You can open it with one hand, at any other time, but not today when it really matters. This time the door will be intransigent until you finally agree to put everything down on the floor and open the door two handed and load yourself up again. All it wanted to do was inconvenience you. You got out of the door in the end and you think you won, but you didn't. You lost. All it wanted to do was inconvenience you.

On the topic of drawers, there is a special thing that is given to screwdrivers. Some are cross-headed and some are flat. Some Human called Phillip, as I understand it, started all that. You keep them all in a 'screwdriver-drawer' cross head and flat headed, all in the drawer together. You need a flat screwdriver today so you go to the drawer, but find that they are all cross-headed. Later, you will need a cross-headed screwdriver so you go to the same drawer knowing that all of yours are cross-headed from your last visit, but No, they are all flat headed. It is given to them to be able to change flat to cross; cross to flat. Not at will. They can only do it if it inconveniences you. They have no power to act; it is your distress that powers it. They cannot prevent you from undoing that screw in the end. They just want to inconvenience you.

Human psychologists will tell you that this is not really happening. It is stress, they say or paranoia, or even schizophrenia. Oh, it is amazing the lengths that you humans will go to just to ignore the obvious truth. Bless you!

Yes. Of course it is stress, and paranoia, and even schizophrenia. That is the way the inanimate operate. They have no will, no ability to act, no real sentience, so they have to wage their war on us by using our own strengths against us. They can use our stress, and paranoia, and even schizophrenia against us. There is a fighting technique invented by pigs, called Ju-Jitsu. I believe that some humans can do it, too. The point of Ju-Jitsu (or Judo) is that small creatures can defeat larger ones by using their opponent's strength against them. That is what the inanimate do. They use our actions and sentience and stress against us.

They want to delay us but they have no ability to do anything, so they use our own actions against us.

Inanimate objects are brilliant team workers. When one thing goes wrong, like a burst pipe, all of the others will join in. That will also be the time that the stop-cock ceases up. That will be when the spanner in the drawer 'hides'. Even unrelated inanimates will join in. That will be the time the door swings shut and strikes your head. That will be the time that the telephone rings. That will be the time that the tea you put on the table jumps off and smashes on the floor.

Don't get me started on things not staying where you put them! You put a pen on a table and it sits there, good as gold. When you turn away it will roll onto the floor. You balance a bucket over the bath and watch to be sure it is stable and only when you turn away will it fall and flood the floor. It will not fall while you watch, because there is greater benefit to wait those few seconds. It can only do it if it inconveniences an Animate. Rodger Rabbit could only get out of handcuffs when it was funny. Inanimates can only do things when it inconveniences an Animate, and only acting through the animate's own actions. The pen does not want to be on the floor. It just wants to be not where you want it to be. It is enough just to inconvenience you. Mind you, if it can spill ink and stain the floor while wrecking its own nib, then so much the better. In the end we will be defeated by attrition. You will always achieve what you set out to do. The action of the inanimate is simply to delay you. If you have been inconvenienced, they are content. Attrition!

New technology plays right into their hands. too. You are putting in a screw in an awkward place. You keep dropping the screw as it wriggles from your hand, dust falls in your eye, the shelf hits you on the head, the door swings shut and you are in the dark. All delaying tactics as the old inanimate teamwork comes into play. However, you persist and finally are ready to screw it in. Here you go. Ready...and... the electric screwdriver is set on undo so it all falls away, crashes on your head and you have to start all over again. Start from scratch. The screwdriver did not set itself to unscrew, of course, you did. - Using your own actions against you. You have one minute before you must deliver a lecture. The hand-outs are locked in a room and you do not have a key, so you decide to quickly photocopy some more; you are not going to be defeated. Then... the photocopier breaks down. It can only do that because you are under pressure. There is a human joke that there is a computer chip in every photocopier to detect when a user is stressed and to have a paper jam just at that moment. Well you can see how the joke starts; they do only jam when you are under extreme pressure. But it is not a computer chip; it is just the inanimate being able to jam at that precise moment because that will cause you the most inconvenience. It can only do it because your distress is what powers the whole process. It can only do it because you are pressed for time. It will use your actions against you – you will feed paper in not squarely and that is at the root of the jam. Using your actions against you. They defeat us by using our actions against us.

There is no fighting back; I know one human who tried. He was walking in a wood, meaning no harm to anyone, when a tree hit him (or so he he said). Naturally being a stout fellow and 'not having

> that', he set to fighting back. He fetched a chain saw and cut
> down the tree. Cut it completely down. That'll teach it!
> It fell on him!
> You can't fight back; you can only try not to mind. If you don't
> mind they can't hurt you.
> More about this another time. If they don't get me first!
> But for now, I can hear a car... Say nothing to Dear Old Neil...
> Good night all of you.
> Elvis.

Appendix 4

There is no appendix 4!

Note: This text is offered on the inventive new 'Createspace' Publishing platform for two reasons:

3) The costs to the reader are far lower than traditional publishing houses.
4) It is easy to update and improve the work; the text is continually under review. To this end the readers and the authors form a community to develop the work. As a reader, you are invited to email suggestions to nwheeler@brookes.ac.uk Contributions may be simple 'typo' alerts, corrections to detail, new areas to cover, etc. All contributors are acknowledged in the print and E-Book versions, and this may be used as material to enhance a CV.

www.ingramcontent.com/pod-product-compliance
Lightning Source LLC
Chambersburg PA
CBHW072133280526
45788CB00002B/620